T0114062

CHAKRADANCE

CHAKRADANCE

MOVE YOUR CHAKRAS, CHANGE YOUR LIFE

NATALIE SOUTHGATE

HAY HOUSE

Carlsbad, California • New York City
London • Sydney • New Delhi

Published in Australia by: Hay House Australia Pty. Ltd.: www.hayhouse.com.au
Published in the United States by: Hay House, Inc.: www.hayhouse.com
Published in the United Kingdom by: Hay House UK, Ltd.: www.hayhouse.co.uk
Published in India by: Hay House Publishers India: www.hayhouse.co.in

Design by Rhett Nacson
Typeset by Bookhouse, Sydney
Edited by Margie Tubbs
Cover photo by Tess Peni
Author photo by Yanni Van Zijl
Illustrations by Stefanie Thompson
Music by Dale Nougher and Natalie Southgate

ISBN: 978-1-4019-6590-7
E-book ISBN: 978-1-4019-5094-1

1st Edition, November 2018

Printed in the United States of America

For Paul, thank you for being on this journey with me.

Thank you for purchasing *Chakradance* by Natalie Southgate.
This product includes 14 free audio downloads.

To access this bonus content,
please visit **www.hayhouse.com.au/download** and enter the
Product ID and **Download Code** as they appear below:

PRODUCT ID: **1934**
DOWNLOAD CODE: **audio**

For further assistance, please contact Hay House Customer Care by phone:
+61 (2) 9669 4299 or visit www.hayhouse.com.au/contact.

Thank you again for your Hay House purchase. Enjoy!

Chakradance Audio Download Track List
> **Base Meditation: Meeting Your Spirit Animal**
> **Move Your Base Chakra**
> **Sacral Meditation: Meet Your Inner Feminine**
> **Move Your Sacral Chakra**
> **Solar Plexus Meditation: Meet Your Inner Masculine**
> **Move Your Solar Plexus Chakra**
> **Heart Meditation: Healing Relationships**
> **Move Your Heart Chakra**
> **Throat Chakra Meditation: Meeting Your Hidden Self**
> **Move Your Throat Chakra**
> **Third Eye Meditation: Awakening Your Intuition**
> **Move Your Third Eye Chakra**
> **Crown Meditation: Soul Message**
> **Move Your Crown Chakra**

CONTENTS

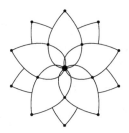

INTRODUCTION

When I was in my mid-twenties, I was living the high life in London. I had a great apartment, ran my own successful recruitment agency and was happily married. From the outside, it all looked perfect and in some ways it was. Yet below the surface, many things were wrong. My health was beginning to deteriorate, as I lived on a diet of fast food, after-work drinks, cigarettes and adrenalin. I was burning the candle at both ends and pushing my body way beyond its limits. But it wasn't just my physical health that was suffering. I felt disconnected—like I was just going through the motions. There was a vague sense of emptiness and no real passion for what I was doing. I was stuck in a life that didn't feel purposeful or authentic to me.

Even though I was aware that my life was way out of balance, I didn't know what to do about it. It was like I was stuck on a treadmill, and I didn't know how to get off.

At that time a woman named Linda worked in the same office building, on the floor below me. Most nights, at five o'clock on the dot, she would run out the door looking excited to be going wherever she was headed. One day I asked her where she went in the evenings. She told me that she worked at The College of Psychic Studies, where they offered courses and training in energy healing, spiritual and psychic development, angels, shamanism, and much more. As she told me about the College, I felt something light up inside me. I couldn't believe such a place existed.

In my late teens and early twenties, I had explored meditation and reiki, but somehow both things had slipped out of my life. Hearing about this College was like a wake-up call. It felt like a part of me that had been sleeping was beginning to stir.

I still vividly remember the day I stepped through the beautiful doors of the College for the first time. I had a sense of coming home. It was a huge turning point in my life. I spent the next five years running my recruitment agency by day and immersing myself in the College by night. I trained as an energy healer and explored all types of intuitive and psychic development. I later went on to teach workshops at the College and work in its clinic as a healer.

It was through my studies that I discovered the chakra system. Finding the map of the chakras was like finding gold for me. For the first time I felt as though I had found a way of looking at life that made complete sense. It was like finding a treasure map to help me navigate my way through life. I really couldn't believe that I hadn't known about this earlier.

The more I dived into the chakras, the more my life began to shift. I began to question whether I was in the right career, the right city, even the right country. I questioned my lifestyle choices, my priorities, my direction. Instead of looking outside myself, I began to look inside for answers. And more importantly, I began to trust my inner voice.

My hunger to know more about the chakras led me to study Jungian psychology and train as a therapist. Carl Jung was one of the first Westerners to work with the Eastern map of the chakras and, although I wasn't particularly drawn to being a therapist, I wanted to know more. The primary aim of Jungian psychology is to form an ongoing relationship between our conscious mind and our unconscious mind. The basic premise is that the more deeply we know ourselves, the richer, fuller and more whole our lives will be. For me, studying Jung was similar to studying the chakras. So much of what I was discovering resonated deeply. I felt like I was waking up more and more each day. I began to feel more passionate and alive than ever before.

It was at this time that I was drawn back to the thing that had always been the key to my happiness as a child: dance. Although the dance classes I took as a child were structured, we were always given time at the end for our own free-form dance. These were the moments I craved the most, when I could just close my eyes and be moved by the music. The sense of freedom I found as I danced was like pure magic.

As I became an adult, dance had somehow disappeared from my life. I instinctively wanted to reconnect with the feeling it had once given me, so I started going to as many different altern-ative dance classes as I could find: shamanic dance, trance dance, improvisation dance, elemental dance and so on. Eventually I found that what I loved doing most was turning off the lights in my own living room, lighting a candle, closing my eyes and dancing. It was as if dance had become my meditation, my healing practice, my way of checking in to see how I was really feeling.

I was thirty years old when I danced a dance that totally changed my life. I had been invited to teach a chakra workshop for beginners at the College that day. When I got home, I lit my candle, cranked up my stereo, closed my eyes and danced. As I moved, I began to experience the music in a whole new way.

Perhaps it was because I'd been working with chakras all day, but I began to feel that different parts of the music were stirring different chakras. I could feel the energy literally pulsing in my body. More than that, I could sense that the images in my mind's eye and the feelings surfacing were directly related to the chakra being stirred by the music.

In that moment, I heard the name 'chakradance' and my instant response was 'yes!' I knew absolutely that I had just found what I needed to create the life I had been yearning for. I needed to dance my chakras. And that was how my life's work and my business was born.

Chakradance

As I explored this new notion that had come to me while dancing, I quickly realised that one of the main keys to Chakradance is the music. Music holds different vibrational frequencies. Just imagine for a moment the difference in feeling between the earthy vibrations of a didgeridoo and the higher vibrations of a lilting flute. Each of our chakras also has its own vibrational frequency. I discovered that if we dance to the right music for each chakra, it balances our energy system. It's like a form of vibrational medicine.

This was one of the most exciting discoveries of my life. The realisation that I could dance my way to a more balanced, passionate and purposeful life was exhilarating for me. It became my mission to find, and later create, the right music for each chakra. Over the years I have spent thousands of hours listening to and **feeling** different musical tracks. Eventually I met a wonderful musician, Dale Nougher, and we now work as a team creating the music for each chakra.

Chakradance began as a practice purely for myself. Each day I would dance a different chakra and then wait to see what would unfold. As well as having insights, emotions and sensations during each dance, I became increasingly mindful of synchronicities, events and happenings in my everyday life. I began to see how dancing a particular chakra would bring to the forefront issues surrounding that chakra. For example, dancing the base chakra might bring up money or safety issues. Dancing the throat chakra might raise communication issues. Specific situations were being brought to my attention to be looked at and healed. It was as though each dance revealed the next step needed on my journey.

As I continued to move my chakras, I began to notice changes in my life. My body felt so much freer, as I began to let go of emotions I had been holding onto. I began to release old patterns that I no longer needed. I became very conscious of which chakras were functioning well and which ones still needed healing. I could also see how all of this was manifesting in my body and in my life. It was as though I began to see life in a whole new way. Dance became the guiding force in my life.

I wasn't the only one who noticed the shifts within me. Friends and colleagues began to ask what I was doing differently. As I began sharing my experiences of Chakradance, I found that others were keen to do it too. The first classes I ever ran were held in my recruitment agency office at night. I'd move the furniture to the sides of the room and cover the desks with brightly-coloured fabrics. I lit candles, burned beautiful oils and transformed my office into a sacred space. I then led others through the practice I'd been doing for myself.

It wasn't long before word spread and I could no longer fit everyone who wanted to learn Chakradance into my office. So I took the plunge and hired a hall for my first official Chakradance workshop. That workshop took place at the Amadeus Centre in Central London. As I guided the group, which included an eighteen-year-old boy and a woman in her late seventies, I knew that this was a practice for everyone.

Soon after, I sold my recruitment business and began what feels like my soul's purpose: to share Chakradance with the world. That was in 2000 and my journey since then has included running workshops all over the world and training hundreds of facilitators to help expand the reach of Chakradance.

I am so excited to be offering this book and the accompanying music. Now you can practise Chakradance in your own home and experience its transformative, healing powers.

Change your life

Having now led thousands of people through the practice of Chakradance, I've discovered that I wasn't alone in feeling stuck in a life that wasn't right for me. So many of us are living lives that feel inauthentic or lacking in passion or real purpose. We may feel stressed out, depressed, addicted or are simply trying to make it through the day—day after day after day.

From my experience, one of the main reasons we feel stuck or stagnant is because we have become disconnected from who we really are and what we really want in our lives. We have become disconnected from our bodies and the wisdom our bodies have to share with us. So many of us are yearning for more. We want more meaning, more soul, more vibrancy in our lives. I truly believe that we can all create the lives we crave. Chakradance can help you get there. It can help you get your life moving again in the right direction.

I am so excited that you are about to embark on your Chakradance journey. As you dance your chakras, you will begin to notice changes in your body and in your life. You may find yourself releasing tension you've been holding onto for years and gaining energy for the things that you want to do in your life. Your dance may put you more in touch with your sensuality and help you reignite your passion. You may find you have more insight into how to handle difficult situations or changes that need to be made in your life.

Working with your chakras can help you to gain more confidence, set boundaries when you need to, and find your authentic voice. You may find more joy in your work, become more connected in your relationships, and wake up each morning looking forward to the day ahead.

When you combine the lessons and insights of this book, the movement of your body, and the healing tones of the music, you will see the transformation in your life. Every time you Chakradance, your energy will shift. Blocks will dissolve and, with practice, you will find freedom, flow and balance in your life.

This is a book to be lived, rather than just read. I encourage you to feel it, breathe it, experience it and dance it. As I write this, I am picturing a snow globe. Everything is already inside the snow globe, but you need to shake it up, to move it, in order to feel the magic and aliveness inside. As you move your chakras, all that is within you will be activated and energised. You will become more awake and alive in your life.

Welcome to Chakradance. Enjoy the journey!

I live a crazy busy life as a single mom with a full-time career in the corporate world. I completely lost my connection to my spiritual inner self, resulting in sickness at one point. So I decided to make drastic changes and started to explore the 'unknown.' I was intuitively drawn to Chakradance, without really knowing anything about it. Chakradance has opened up a new world for me and my healing journey snowballed after that. The 'unknown' turned out to be my homecoming. I feel truly blessed with the abundance that I experience in my life now. My life has changed in so many wonderful ways.

Caroline

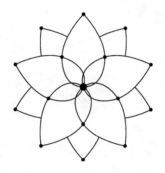

PART 1

The ELEMENTS
OF CHAKRADANCE

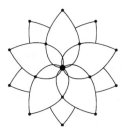

CHAPTER ONE

WHAT is CHAKRADANCE?

At its core, Chakradance is a fusion of four key elements: the chakras, dance, music and mandala art—a creative art making process that acts as a bridge between our inner and outer worlds. Each of these four elements has its own healing power, but it is the way they are used, as well as the way in which they are woven together, that creates the healing power of Chakradance.

On this journey, I will guide you into a dance for each of your chakras. I'll begin with the base chakra (located at the base of your spine) and move all the way up to your crown chakra (at the top of your head).

Before you start dancing, you will benefit from having a basic knowledge of how and why Chakradance works. The following chapters focus on each of the four elements mentioned above.

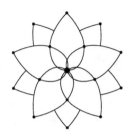

CHAPTER TWO

the FIRST ELEMENT—
the CHAKRAS

Shortly after I began Chakradance, I felt drawn to India. I was eager to learn as much about the chakras as I could so travelling to the place where they were discovered felt like something I needed to do. My husband and I filled our backpacks and left our comfortable lives in search of ancient wisdom. We spent five months on this quest. We visited temples, undertook various Ayurvedic therapies, and spent time engaging with the local children. We danced on beaches, endured intense bouts of sickness, and witnessed some incredible sights.

Although I learnt a lot on this adventure, the biggest thing I absorbed was that to understand my chakras, I needed to look inside. It wasn't India that I needed to travel to after all; it was the journey within that was calling.

Our chakras are a very real part of who we are. They are not separate from us. They don't live outside of us. They are us. We are more than just physical bodies. Surrounding us is a dynamic, electromagnetic energy field commonly known as the aura. Our aura is like a matrix containing our mental, emotional and spiritual energies, all of which interconnect with our physical body.

The role of the chakras is to help regulate the flow of energy in and out of our auras and bodies. When this energy flows freely, we feel healthy, vibrant and balanced. When the flow is blocked, our health and wellbeing reflect this imbalance.

The word 'chakra' originates from Sanskrit, the ancient language of India, and translates as 'wheel.' We can picture the chakras as pulsing wheels or vortexes of energy in our auras.

There are seven major chakras, which are outlined in the diagram that follows. These seven chakras align from the base of the spinal column, progressing upward to the crown of the head. On a physical level, the chakras correlate with specific organs, nerve ganglia and the endocrine system—the collection of glands that regulate physiological processes by releasing hormones. On a nonphysical level, each of the chakras directly influences a specific aspect of our lives, from our primal instincts to our spirituality. Together, the seven chakras encompass the whole of human experience, and can therefore act as a map to guide us through life.

Carl Jung believed that the map of the chakras mirrored what he named 'The Process of Individuation.' He likened this process to a spiritual quest in search of a sense of wholeness and depth in our lives. He believed that each chakra serves as a kind of stepping stone on our soul's journey through life.

As I've studied the chakras, I have found that every issue or problem we face in life can be directly linked to a chakra. For example, grief is related to the heart chakra, digestive issues to the solar plexus chakra, and lack of imagination to the third eye chakra. Whether the issue is physical, emotional, mental or spiritual, balancing our chakras is key to finding balance and wellbeing in our lives.

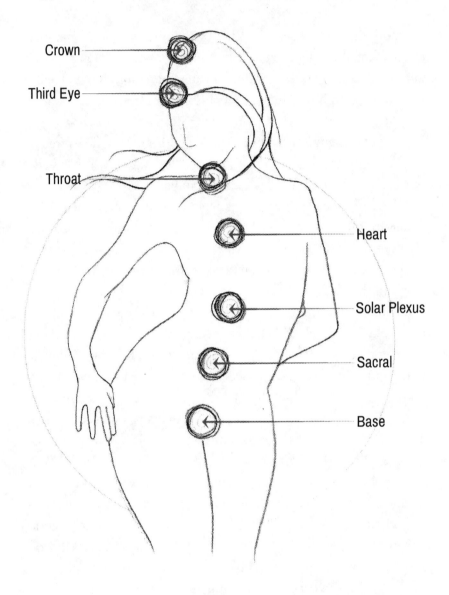

Balancing the chakras

As we journey through our lives, our chakras can become out of balance. There are all kinds of reasons for this. Everything affects our chakras—from the food we eat and the toxins we breathe to the shocks, traumas and emotions we experience. The family we grew up in and the events that take place in our lives—some even say our past lives—all have an impact on our chakras. The aim of Chakradance is to rebalance our chakras and bring them into a state of vibrancy and health.

All chakra imbalances are the result of stuck energy. Through Chakradance, we begin to dislodge the blockages by moving the energy in our chakras. As we release this trapped energy, we transform our health and our lives. As we dance each chakra, it's as though we shine a spotlight on a specific area of our lives. As the energy moves, it can cause old memories to surface, as well as a variety of feelings, sensations, images, insights and even a heightened awareness into situations in our lives.

Chakradance is not just about what happens during the dance. As we step into our lives afterwards, it's as though we experience the world through the lens of the chakra we've just danced. Issues directly relating to a chakra tend to present themselves, so we can transform them. For example, dancing the heart chakra may immediately bring to the forefront a relationship that needs healing. Issues around our sexual lives may surface after dancing the sacral chakra. After dancing the throat chakra, we may find ourselves needing to finally speak our truth.

In many ways, our outer lives are a reflection of our chakras. Just take a moment to reflect on your own life. What parts are flowing and where do you feel blocked? For example, perhaps you are stuck in a job that bores you, and yet you haven't done anything about it. This indicates that you may have an imbalanced solar plexus chakra, and are lacking the confidence to ask for a promotion, or apply for a new job that is far more stimulating. Or maybe you are in a relationship where you feel perpetually jealous, needy and possessive? Although it's easy to blame your partner, these symptoms indicate an imbalance in your heart chakra and the underlying need for self-love.

To share an example from my own life, I used to be extremely uncomfortable with public speaking. My throat would go dry, my hands would sweat, and I would literally feel sick to my stomach whenever I had to get up in front of a group of people. On one occasion, I even lost my voice completely. I had noticed various symptoms and signs suggesting that both my throat chakra and my solar plexus chakra were imbalanced, so I began dancing them (the throat chakra for authentic expression and the solar plexus chakra for confidence and personal power) before any public speaking engagement. The difference was profound. As I've continued to dance these chakras and bring them into a more balanced state, I no longer experience any negative issues with public speaking. Sure, I still get nervous, but I now associate the feeling with excitement rather than terror.

Even though we will explore each of our chakras individually on this journey, it's helpful to remember that each chakra is connected to the others. Together they form a system, so a blockage in one chakra will impact on the others.

The good news is that balancing one chakra has a positive impact on the whole. For example, if we have blocked energy at the base chakra, we might find ourselves becoming overly concerned with the material aspects of our lives. We might find ourselves hoarding possessions, holding onto excess weight, or having extreme feelings of tiredness and heaviness. This imbalance in the base chakra may make it difficult for us to engage with the higher chakras. We may struggle to connect with our higher self and find it difficult to trust our intuition or see the bigger picture. As we balance the base chakra and begin to release the blockages, energy is freed up to flow to the higher chakras. Moving one chakra creates movement in the others.

When we Chakradance, we are consciously interacting with our chakras and choosing to balance our energy. As we dance, we literally change our energy in a positive way. We become more energetically healthy and, when we are energetically healthy, it's like we vibrate at a different frequency. This new frequency or vibration can attract wonderful new situations, opportunities and people into our lives.

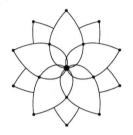

CHAPTER THREE

the SECOND ELEMENT—
DANCE

Just as chakra wisdom can be traced back many thousands of years, so too can the healing power of dance. In ancient times, dance featured at the heart of many celebrations and rituals. People danced the shifting of the seasons, the waxing and waning of the moon, as well as life's great transitions like birth, death and coming into womanhood. Our ancestors danced to connect to the spirit world, to go into altered states of consciousness, and to find meaning in their lives.

Hindus are still taught their great epics through dance, and the Sufi whirling dervishes spin in search of enlightenment. Clubbing culture is a massive worldwide phenomenon, where dancers enter a trance-like state due to the hypnotic effect of repetitive beats and movements. From ancient temples to modern nightclubs, dance remains a powerful method of connecting to our own sacredness. I would argue that the need for dance as a way of healing is stronger than ever these days.

We are born to dance and move freely. We only have to look at young children and watch their natural movements when they hear music to believe this. The freedom of expression they display is innate in all of us. Sadly, as our energy becomes blocked for all the reasons I mentioned previously, from unhealthy living to traumatic experiences, so too does our freedom of movement.

We hold our blocked emotions and mental challenges in both our physical bodies and our chakras. This trapped energy causes tension and tightness in our bodies. It keeps us stuck in negative patterns that stop us from moving forward in our lives.

The physical movement of Chakradance keeps our energy moving and flowing. It is therefore a safe way to release buried or bottled-up feelings and unhealthy patterns. As we dance each chakra, we cleanse our bodies of trapped trauma and tension. We can let go of negative thoughts, as we open up to higher levels of consciousness. Healing takes place within our energy fields and within the very cells of our bodies.

Chakradance is a free-form, spontaneous dance that takes on a different expression with each chakra. The dance of each chakra will be unique to each of us and may well be different every time we dance. How we dance our chakras has much more to do with our energy and how it's flowing than with our talent or expertise. We don't need to worry about what we look like, or whether we are doing it right, as we Chakradance. Our only task is to simply allow the dance to unfold and to notice the sensations and emotions that surface and move through our bodies; to notice the images, intuitions and inspirations that arise from our souls. When we surrender ourselves fully to the dance, we can let go of trying to dance in a certain way, trying to make something specific happen, trying to control our feelings or reactions. We simply become moving energy. Chakradance is not a **doing**. It's an **undoing**, a letting go.

Chakradance is most powerful when we dance in darkness. Whether we close our eyes, wear an eye mask or dance in a darkened room, the darkness helps us turn our attention inward. In this internal space, it can feel like we are dancing in a waking dream. We may see, hear, smell and taste things that have previously been hidden from us. We may meet aspects of ourselves that we have forgotten. Buried feelings or repressed memories may surface. We may open up to alternate realities or encounter loved ones who have crossed over.

Chakradance takes us deep inside ourselves. It reveals our darkness, our pain and our wounds, but it also leads us to the beauty, the bliss and the freedom in our lives. It helps us to experience all that we are. We may not always intellectually understand what is happening in our dance, but there is always great healing going on as we move the energy of our chakras. Chakradance is not something that's meant to be analysed or overthought; focus instead on being in the moment and let the experience unfold.

Much like meditation, Chakradance is a practice. The more committed we stay to the practice, the deeper the benefits. Each dance is a step towards more freedom in our lives. With each dance, we release the next blockage and allow more energy to flow. Dance by dance, we move our way to wholeness and find a greater sense of balance in our lives.

Dances of the chakras

– BASE CHAKRA

The dance of the base chakra connects us to our primal, instinctual energy. It helps us to reclaim the wild, animal-like part of us and deepens our connection to the earth. We may find ourselves emphasising movements of our legs and feet in this tribal, raw, primitive dance.

— SACRAL CHAKRA

Dancing the sacral chakra deepens our connection with our sacred feminine energy, which is innate within both women and men. Like water, our feelings and sensuality flow from this chakra. Fluid, sensual movements of our hips and belly can heighten our sense of pleasure and passion.

— SOLAR PLEXUS CHAKRA

As we dance the solar plexus chakra, we express our inner masculine energy. This fiery energy fuels our dance, helping us to feel confident and strong. We may find ourselves doing dynamic martial arts movements, as we rediscover our own warrior power.

— HEART CHAKRA

We use our breath to expand our chest and lift up into the airy dance of the heart chakra. This soft and gentle dance opens us up to love, kindness and compassion for others, but also for ourselves. This dance, which may call us to whirl and soar, can help us open up to the lightness and joy within us.

— THROAT CHAKRA

The throat chakra helps us to express our authentic truth. The dance of the throat chakra is a mantra dance, where we weave together our voice and movements. The vibrations of the sounds we create pulse through our bodies, intensifying our self-expression and creativity. We become moving sound.

— THIRD EYE CHAKRA

As we surrender into a trance dance, we may find ourselves making hypnotic and repetitive movements. We may also open ourselves up to visions, insights and higher guidance from our third eye chakra. This dance heightens our perceptions and helps us see the bigger picture.

– CROWN CHAKRA

The dance of the crown chakra feels like a dancing prayer. We may find ourselves raising our arms towards the sky, to receive the light of universal love, grace and wisdom. This is the dance of our soul.

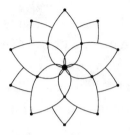

CHAPTER FOUR

the THIRD ELEMENT— MUSIC

We have all experienced the powerful effects of music. Who doesn't remember a time when hearing an old song caused them to become flooded with raw emotion for a person, place or period in their lives? Music has a way of instantly transporting us back, so once again we feel just as we did all those years ago. Or perhaps we wake up depressed, but when we hear our favourite song playing on the radio, our mood is lifted by the familiar tune. The magic of music lies in its unique capacity to touch us on many different levels—physically, emotionally and spiritually—making it a powerful tool for healing.

For centuries, cultures around the world have used music to create balance and healing. In ancient times, music played the role of healer and therapist. It was a vital tonic for the body, mind and spirit in the ancient cultures of Egypt, Greece, India and China. Tibetan Buddhists used (and still use) bowls, chimes and bells, creating tones and vibrations to enhance spiritual practice. Shamans in both Native American and Australian Aboriginal communities used repetitive sound (for example, chanting or sacred drumming) and vocal toning (the sustained singing of certain notes) to create a sense of balance and harmony. Music in many cultures has been composed and performed with the intention of freeing one's emotions, entering into altered states of consciousness and, ultimately, healing the soul.

Music has also been shown to have a profound physiological effect on us. There is more research on music than any other creative healing modality. It has been shown to help reduce physical pain, alleviate stress, clear our thinking and elevate our mood. It can soothe or awaken our nervous system, arouse passion and bring us into deep states of peace. In his book *Music and Miracles*, Don Campbell, director of the Institute for Music, Health and Education in Boulder, Colorado, shares stories of how he has seen many unexplained, miraculous events associated with music. He has seen Alzheimer patients who could not be reached in any other way respond clearly to questions asked through song. He has even seen comatose patients regain awareness through response to music.

Music can have such a profound physical, mental and spiritual effect on us because we don't just hear it with our ears—we feel its vibrations in our bodies and in our auras. The energetic waves of music literally pulse through us. Even people who have lost their sense of hearing can feel the beat and pulsing of music within their bodies. Music can create vibrational shifts in our bodies and our energy fields. Where we have stuck or blocked energy, physically or energetically, the vibrations of sound can dislodge those blockages, clearing the way for new, healthier patterns to flow. So is it any wonder that music plays a major role in Chakradance?

In the early days of Chakradance, I met a beautiful soul named Susie, a sound healer who introduced me to the incredible power and beauty of quartz crystal bowls. When these unique instruments are played, they create clear vibrational soundwaves, with each bowl pulsing a specific tone. Whenever I would meet with Susie to play the bowls, I would intuitively start feeling which bowl resonated with each chakra. Susie sourced bowls from all over the world and it took many months before I found a set of bowls that felt vibrationally right. These bowls have formed the backbone of all our Chakradance music since then.

Later I met musician, Dale Nougher, and together we have created music that resonates with each of the seven chakras. Each track is a fusion of modern dance music blending specific instruments and rhythms that activate each chakra—from grounding, tribal beats and sounds for the base chakra to more ethereal, expansive music for the higher chakras—interwoven with the vibrational tones of chakra crystal bowls.

These tracks are such an important part of the Chakradance experience that we are making them available to you to download. You'll find instructions for how to do this on page vi. As you dance to the healing music created for each chakra, allow yourself to really feel it. Feel the vibrations in the pores of your skin, in the pulsing energy field around you. Let the rhythms, beats and tones dance through you.

When I first heard the beautiful, powerful music of Chakradance, I felt like I had come home. Tears streamed down my face. For once I felt alive and not like I was just going through the motions.

Nadine

Music of the chakras

– BASE CHAKRA

The music for the base chakra resonates with the frequency of red (the most dense of the seven-colour spectrum). The music is earthy, raw and primal. Didgeridoos, tribal beats and chants call us to connect with our instincts, our land and our ancestors.

– SACRAL CHAKRA

The music for the sacral chakra resonates with the frequency of orange. The voices of goddesses and the gentle sounds of the ocean open us to our feelings and our innate feminine energy. The sensual, smouldering Middle Eastern rhythms flood us with pleasure and passion.

– SOLAR PLEXUS CHAKRA

Solar plexus music vibrates to the colour yellow. The chants of spiritual warriors over the sounds of a roaring fire call forth our inner masculine energy. The beats and rhythms of the solar plexus are strong, powerful, driving and dynamic.

– HEART CHAKRA

The music of the heart chakra vibrates to the colour green. Lilting flutes like the whispers of angels interweave with the heartbeat of sacred drums. These soaring sounds open our hearts to lightness and love.

– THROAT CHAKRA

The music for the throat chakra vibrates to the colour sky blue. A distinctly intense humming vibration weaves together with the ethereal sounds of a spiritual choir. This calls us to become part of a ceremony of sound, to dance to the greater rhythm of life.

— THIRD EYE CHAKRA

The music of the third eye chakra vibrates to the colour indigo, the colour of the night sky. High vibrational frequencies mixed with repetitive, hypnotic beats take us on a trance-like journey into higher realms.

— CROWN CHAKRA

The music for the crown chakra vibrates to the colour violet, the highest and fastest vibration in the seven-colour spectrum. Heavenly voices and sounds weave in and out through the beat of the music. Here we experience a heaven on earth.

Guided imagery

When we Chakradance, we go on an inner journey. Dancing the seven chakras is like dancing our way into seven different inner worlds, each with its own lessons, stories and gifts.

Each of the Chakradance tracks includes guided visualisations, in the form of spoken words woven throughout the music. These visualisations are there to help lead you inward and point you towards the gifts of each chakra. Having experienced the guided imagery in your dance, you can then take the learnings and gifts into your daily life.

For example, for the base chakra we visualise being in a tropical jungle, with our feet dancing on soft red mud. Our ancestors or spirit animals may join us in our dance. This might evoke feelings of stability and security or a powerful physical sensation of being present in your body. After your dance, if you are faced with a challenging situation, the gifts from the base chakra will help you to stand your ground, trust your instincts, and deal with what is happening more effectively.

By contrast, when dancing the heart chakra we visualise a magnificent angel asking us to hand over anything that is weighing down our hearts, before we breathe in the light from the angel. This dance may evoke feelings and sensations of compassion and love. After dancing the heart chakra, you may find that you are a little more kind and gentle with yourself and others.

The guided visualisations in Chakradance help us to dance the healing gifts from our chakras out into our lives; we dance the sensations of the imagery into our reality. Feel free to follow the guidance I offer you with the music, or allow your imagination to take you on your own inner journey. As you dance deeper into your inner worlds, be open to the feelings, sensations and memories that unfold.

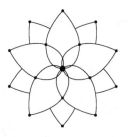

CHAPTER FIVE

the FOURTH ELEMENT— MANDALA ART

When we dance each chakra, it can feel like we are in a waking dream. Our experiences often feel like they take place beyond time or space. Our feelings and sensitivity can be heightened and we may find that energy and insights are flowing through us. In Chakradance, we anchor this energy by creating a mandala after our dance.

When I began studying Jungian psychology in the late 1990s, part of my training involved undergoing personal therapy. Over the following decade, I worked with two amazing Jungian analysts, who both had an enormous influence in my life. Sally, the therapist I was with for most of those years, introduced me to the idea of working with art, as a way of anchoring the powerful energy that would often surface during our sessions.

Because my Chakradance experiences also released powerful energies, I decided to try creating art after I danced. Through my studies of Jung, I had discovered the concept of mandala art making—the process of spontaneously drawing or painting inside a circle. I felt drawn to try this process after dance and couldn't believe what began to happen! Creating a mandala not only grounded the energy of my dance, it also created a kind of bridge between my inner and outer worlds. It felt like a creative expression of the energy of the chakra I had just danced—a visual representation of my inner landscape. Not only could I see and feel the energy as I created the art, but throughout the process I continued to receive more insight and guidance into the chakra I had just danced.

An example of this is when I danced the sacral chakra shortly after the birth of my second child. In my dance, I experienced feelings of loss and sadness. On a purely intellectual level this made no sense to me, as I was delighted to be a mother and felt very happy in my daily life. In my mandala, I spontaneously drew a mask. As I was creating this mask I continued to feel loss and sadness weighing me down. I gained the insight that, with my mother role dominating so heavily at that time, I had lost (or masked) the sensual, wild and passionate part of myself, and this was causing me some inner pain. My mandala gave me the guidance to have some fun, spend time with my girlfriends, and give myself time to play. This was an invaluable message for me at that time.

Mandalas have been used in the ancient cultures of Buddhism and Hinduism for thousands of years. However, Carl Jung is credited with introducing this Eastern concept to Western thought. In 1916, he began creating his own mandala paintings by drawing shapes that corresponded to how he was feeling in the moment. He believed that the images were rising spontaneously from his inner world, almost like sacred symbols containing messages for him. He believed that mandalas symbolise 'a safe refuge of inner reconciliation and wholeness.'

Mandala is a Sanskrit word that translates as 'magic circle.' The circle is a universal symbol of wholeness and totality. When used in a mandala, it becomes the container, or holder, of our experience.

In Chakradance, we create a mandala after we dance by drawing our experience inside a circle. The drawing can be abstract, using colours, patterns or shapes to reflect our inner feelings, moods or energy. Or we may draw literal, vivid images that represent our visions from the dance.

Initially, I felt hesitant about creating a mandala because I've always thought of myself as someone who can't draw. But then I realised, just as we don't need to be professional dancers to dance our chakras, we don't need to consider ourselves artists to create a mandala. Our mandala is a pure expression of our energy. We don't plan what we are going to draw. Much like our dance, it's an intuitive process that unfolds spontaneously.

I have been creating mandalas for many years now. When I look back on them, some do look quite pleasing but many could be described as unattractive. What they all have in common is that they are pulsing with energy. Each one is a raw expression of whatever was going on for me in that chakra at that time. They are like an outward, visual representation of my inner life. I've found it interesting to look back at my mandalas and notice the themes that often resurface around a particular chakra. The mandalas often serve as a record of the subtle healings that have taken place dance by dance.

Shortly after I began creating my own mandala art, I introduced it into my Chakradance classes and found the feedback reflected my own experiences. Now mandala art is an important feature of every Chakradance class. I encourage you to try creating your own mandalas after you have danced each of the chakras, so that you too can experience their power and insight.

How to create a mandala

To create a mandala, all you need is a piece of paper with a circle drawn on it. You may want to buy yourself a book with blank pages, so that you can keep all your mandalas together. I personally use black paper, because I find colours pop against this background and the black feels like it represents the inner world I have just experienced. However, you can choose whatever colour paper you wish. To draw the 'magic circle' in which you will create your mandala, I suggest tracing the outline of a dinner plate or something of similar size.

You will also need some pastels to draw with. Oil pastels or soft pastels both work well and are easy to use. You will want to have your art materials fully prepared and placed nearby before you dance.

I recommend creating your mandala immediately after you dance. As you finish dancing, take three slow, deep breaths and then sit with your art materials in front of you. Place your non-dominant hand into the centre of the circle and imagine pouring the energy of the chakra you have just danced into that circle. Spend a few minutes filling the circle energetically before using your pastels to creatively express the mood, feelings and imagery from your dance. Let go of any expectations about what will emerge. Just let your creativity flow.

When you have finished your mandala, spend a few minutes reflecting on it (but not judging it). After that, write the answers to the following questions next to your mandala:

- What is the name (or title) of your mandala?
- What feelings do you have when you look at your mandala?
- What question is your mandala asking of you?

Try not to think too hard about the answers. Just go with the first thoughts that come to you.

Our mandalas can provide us with wonderful insight, wisdom and guidance. You may want to hang your mandala where you can see it or keep it in a safe place. Your mandala is a sacred representation of your inner world and you can return to it to connect with this energy whenever you need to.

The privilege of a lifetime is to
become who you truly are.
Who looks outside, dreams; who looks inside, awakes.

Carl Jung, Swiss psychiatrist and psychoanalyst

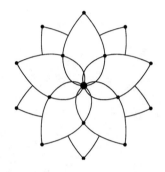

PART 2

PREPARING for YOUR JOURNEY

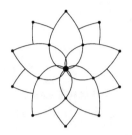

CHAPTER SIX

the ADVENTURE AHEAD

When I was twenty and getting ready to go backpacking around Europe, I bought a guidebook called *Let's Go* that became my map and travelling companion. It led me to great destinations, from major cities to villages I'd never heard of, and kept me on course through highs and lows. Sometimes I was terrified and felt so out of my depth in foreign places, and other times I revelled in the new delights I had found. The whole experience was an adventure; one that helped me discover a lot about myself and grow as a person.

Move your Chakras, Change your Life with Chakradance is also a kind of guidebook, except that it is a guide for the most profound journey any of us will ever take—the journey within. It invites us into the unknown wilderness of our own being. On this adventure we will discover our true, authentic self, which will ultimately lead us to a life of freedom, flow and balance.

I didn't write this book because I have all the answers to life, but because I've been fortunate to discover some really great tools that can help any of us on our life's journey. I believe this journey is ultimately about remembering who we truly are, and then connecting with others and the world from this place of truth.

Life can be fragile and fleeting in the grand scheme of things. It is sacred and meant to be lived and embraced to the fullest. The day I began writing this book was my mother's seventy-first birthday. When I wished her a happy birthday, she said: 'The only advice I have for you is to really live your life; live it as fully as you can, as it goes by so quickly.'

That same day I stumbled across a book called *The Top Five Regrets of the Dying* by Bronnie Ware, a carer who worked with people in palliative care. The regrets touch upon being more genuine, not working so hard, expressing one's true feelings, staying in touch with friends and finding more joy in life.

I took these messages as signs to keep writing this book. That's because it is a book about truly living, about feeling, remembering, discovering and expressing all that we truly are. In this book I share with you all I have discovered on my own journey so far, as well as some insights from the beautiful souls who have graciously contributed their stories to this book.

As you embark on the journey into your own chakras, be open to the changes within you—to feeling more alive, fully present and free.

As with any journey we undertake, planning needs to be done ahead of time so we can get the most out of the experience. The following preparations will help you get ready for your dancing adventure, which will begin in Part 3 of this book when you dance your base chakra. In addition, you may intuitively find your own ways of preparing for your journey.

Envisioning your journey

This book is a journey of seven steps, with each of the following sections guiding you into one of the seven chakras. If you would like to get the most from this book, I encourage you to dedicate one week to each step, in order to really engage in each chakra's dance, meditation and accompanying exercises. And that's just to start with. Once you've made your way through all seven chakras, I recommend returning to each of the dances regularly to really get the most of out of them.

If you are anything like me, you may want to read through the whole book first, so that you know what the journey is about, and then schedule your seven weeklong sessions, one for each chakra. However, if you feel drawn to diving straight in, then please go ahead. There is no right or wrong way to approach this journey, only the way that feels right for you.

You are likely to find that you feel more comfortable in some chakras than others. Your movements may be natural and at ease in some dances but stilted or awkward in others. Some of the music may really resonate with you and some may not. You may find yourself easily surrendering into some exercises but becoming distracted in others. Some chakras may even surprise you. Take notice of your differing responses, because they are clues to which of your chakras are healthy and which need balancing.

When I first began dancing the base chakra, I used to find the music very irritating. I'd struggle to find the right movements in my body, and I felt awkward and uncoordinated. I would often find myself distracted in the dance and start thinking about what I was going to have for dinner later that night, or what shopping needed to be done. My feelings, thoughts and sensations were all indicators of the imbalance I had in my base chakra. My experiences in the dance were simply mirroring the way my base chakra was functioning in my life at that time. As I've continued on my

Chakradance journey, my base chakra has become far more balanced. I now find myself surrendering freely to the tribal beats and grounding moves. I am now far more comfortable in my own body and that is reflected in my dance.

As you focus on a particular chakra, it helps to take note of what is happening in your daily life. The issues surrounding each chakra are often brought to our attention during and after our dance, so they can be resolved. As you move your chakras, you will gain a clearer sense of how your energy system is functioning and how this impacts on your health and your life. As blocked energy begins to flow more freely, you will notice corresponding shifts and changes in your life.

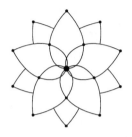

CHAPTER SEVEN

PRACTICAL PREPARATION— MUSIC and MANDALA ART

Downloading the music

I recommend that you begin by downloading the seven Chakradance tracks and seven chakra meditations included with this book onto a device (iPod, iPad, computer, etc.) that will be easily accessible for you to play them on, wherever and whenever you choose to dance. (refer to page vi)

While doing this, think about how you might best play the music at a high volume, especially for the dances, where you want to be able to really **feel** the music, not just hear it.

Preparing to create your mandala art

Prepare paper and pastels for your mandala art, as suggested on page 24. I would recommend having the circle traced and the packet of pastels opened before you begin, so that you are ready to create your mandala art immediately after dancing.

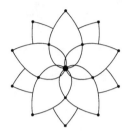

CHAPTER EIGHT

CREATING a SACRED SPACE

Creating your own space where you can dance and practise your meditations and reflections is a way of honouring the sacredness of what you are doing. It is a way of honouring the deeper part of yourself that you will be connecting with on this journey.

Creating a sacred space really just means preparing a safe space where you feel nurtured and completely comfortable letting go. I've found it's helpful to physically clean the space first. When we tidy up, it shifts the old, stuck energy in the space. We can then bring into the space anything that feels sacred or meaningful for us. I like to light a candle (to symbolically bring in light) and burn essential oils (to infuse the space). I also have a beautiful sculpture of an ancient goddess that a close friend gave to me at a particularly challenging time in my life. For me the goddess symbolises strength and power and serves as a reminder of what I have inside. Finally, I have a set of chimes that I ring at the beginning and end of my dance or sacred work, which helps in the 'holding' of the experience for me.

When I studied Jungian psychology, I learnt a lot about the concept of 'holding.' It refers to a safe container where we can unfold our inner world. Creating a sacred space is like creating our very own container, almost like a womb, where we can birth new parts of ourselves safely.

The other wonderful thing about creating a sacred space is that it helps us surrender more quickly into our experiences. Our space holds the energy and sacredness of previous energy work. Over time this continues to build, and we start to feel the difference the minute we arrive in the space. Our sacred space becomes our safe haven, a special place we can retreat to whenever we feel the need to create a sense of calm and peace or want to simply spend time with ourselves.

Most of us won't have a spare room to set up especially for this purpose, but that's okay. A sacred space can be set up in the corner of the bedroom or living room. It can be a space in the garden or on the back porch. It doesn't matter where it is or how big it is, as long as it feels safe and nurturing and there is enough room to dance without bumping into anything.

If you spend time travelling and staying in hotel rooms or as a guest in other people's houses, you can still create a sacred space wherever you are staying. Simply bring into the space one or more of the objects or rituals that are meaningful to you in your own sacred space at home, like lighting a candle or imagining filling the room with light. You can also create a sacred space within that is available wherever you go. I see my inner sacred space as a clearing in a forest. There is a beautiful waterfall flowing into a sparkling river. A rainbow of colours dance in the reflection of the water. I can smell the perfume of exotic flowers. Whenever I close my eyes and go to this space, I feel at peace and relaxed.

Experiment with creating your own sacred space, both in the outer world and within, so that there will always be sacred space available to you when you want or need it.

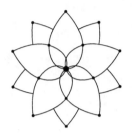

CHAPTER NINE

SETTING an INTENTION

Setting a clear intention each time I dance, meditate or carry out an exercise, helps to energise and fuel my commitment. You can do the same by taking a moment before beginning each activity to let go of all the things that have been going on throughout your day. Then consciously set an intention to fully surrender to your dance or meditation and be open to the messages and insights it has for you. You may like to say something simple like: *I let go of all that has happened today. I am fully present here in my sacred space. I am open to the insight and guidance my dance has for me.*

Setting an intention isn't just a superficial act. When we do this, we are communicating with our inner world and preparing ourselves to start something new. I like to see the intention I am setting as a laser beam of focused energy sending a very clear message that I am here in this moment and ready to commit to the work that needs to be done.

After setting your intention, let it go. This allows you to be fully present in your practice, while trusting that your inner world will respond. We don't need to force anything or try too hard. It's like throwing a fishing line out into the sea. Like a fisherman, we stay calm and committed, waiting for what comes.

While it may seem contradictory, letting go of expectations is an important aspect of intention setting. Sometimes our conscious mind has a fixed idea of what it thinks will or should happen, but our inner world has other ideas. Staying open and allowing the dance or meditation to simply unfold allows for more spontaneity and grace in the process.

Setting an intention doesn't just work in our sacred space as we prepare to dance. Setting an intention as you wake each morning is also a great habit to start practising. The intention you set could be something like being more fully present in each moment, bringing an open heart to every exchange you have throughout the day, or whatever has meaning for you in that moment.

The simplest way to set an intention is to close your eyes and take three slow, deep breaths. With each breath, become increasingly more present in the moment. From this place of centred calm, recite either silently or out loud a simple positive statement of intention. Finish by again taking three deep breaths and opening your eyes. That's it. Then proceed with your dance, meditation or your day.

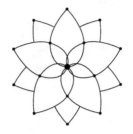

CHAPTER TEN

CLEANSING YOUR ENERGY FIELD

Every day, we absorb different energies into our energy fields. When we spend time with other people, it is unavoidable that we literally take on some of their energy, both positive and negative. Likewise, fragments of the energy from places we visit can get absorbed into our fields. And of course, our own thought patterns and emotions can also cause our energy fields to become heavy and dense.

Just as our physical bodies need to be cleaned, stretched and exercised, so too do our auras need looking after. To maintain good energetic health we need to cleanse our field daily just as we shower our physical bodies or brush our teeth. The clearer our energy field, the more alive, energised and vibrant we feel.

Before you dance, meditate or carry out one of the exercises in this book, it is a good idea to spend a couple minutes cleansing your energy field. Below are a couple of visualisations that work for me. After you have done them a few times, you may find that your own visualisations start to come to you. Feel free to let your imagination guide you towards what you most need.

– CLEANSING WITH WHITE LIGHT

Stand relaxed with your feet planted firmly on the ground. Soften your breath and imagine a white light washing all over you like a waterfall. Visualise the light dissolving all unwanted energies. Imagine this light moving through every part of your physical body and your entire energy body. Continue to visualise the light pouring over you until you feel completely cleansed. You may intuitively feel like changing the colour of the light on different days or at different times. Trust whatever feels right for you.

In addition to doing this before you dance or meditate, it's a great idea to do this exercise in the shower, where you can use the running water as part of your visualisation. This can then become part of your daily cleansing ritual, where both your physical and energy bodies are purified.

I also use this visualisation as I walk through my front door. Part of my daily routine for years has been to visualise a stream of white light shining right through me and around me just before I step inside my door. My intention is to release anything that is not mine or not needed before I step into my home.

– RELEASING NEGATIVE ENERGY

Sit quietly and take three slow, deep breaths. Visualise a mesh door made out of light in front of you. See yourself walking through the door and imagine all the unwanted energies attached to you being filtered out as you move through the mesh. These unwanted energies may be your fears, worries, tiredness, negative thought patterns, stuck emotions, etc.

Next, see yourself standing on the other side of the door feeling cleansed and purified. You may then want to walk through another door, made of finer mesh. Continue this visualisation until you see your energy field shining a pure white light.

These techniques are most powerful when we repeat them often. I recommend experimenting with the exercises and finding a daily practice that is simple and easy to stick to. It can help to choose regular times to practise each day, like when you first wake up in the morning or during the last few minutes of the day before you go to sleep. Then, with time, they will become a natural part of your daily routine. These exercises don't need to take a lot of time. Just a few minutes on a regular basis can yield incredible results.

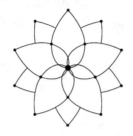

CHAPTER ELEVEN

JOURNALLING

I encourage you to keep a journal as you work with your chakras. You may wish to record any inspirations that come to you after you dance or note any synchronicities, chance encounters, experiences or events that surface during your day, which you feel are connected to the chakra you are exploring. When working with the chakras, it is common to have a more active dream life than usual. Recording any dreams, memories or feelings that surface during the night also helps with the process.

As I was writing this book and journeying through my own chakras, I began having dreams of my clothes not fitting me anymore. They all seemed to be the wrong colours or sizes. I then dreamt that, as I looked at myself in the mirror, it smashed into pieces. As I was journalling about these dreams and the feelings that came with them, I had the insight that some old ways of being were no longer fitting me. It was time to let these old ways go, as a new reflection was forming. I took this as an encouraging sign of growth in my life. Journalling about it helped me make sense of what was happening and made me aware of the small shifts that were taking place in my daily life.

Committing to a few minutes of journalling every morning and night helps to build the connection between our inner and outer worlds. It helps bridge our unconscious and our consciousness. The more these two aspects of ourselves are in communication, the more whole and balanced we become.

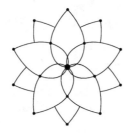

CHAPTER TWELVE

FINDING YOUR RHYTHM

As you start this journey, I encourage you to find a rhythm that works for you. Our inner world responds well to rhythms and repetitions. For example, you may choose to dance one chakra at the beginning of each week and engage in the exercises for that chakra throughout the rest of the week. Or you may choose to dance every morning and do your reflections and reading in the evenings. You may need to experiment in the beginning to find what works best for you. Then when you find a rhythm, commit to it.

When I was in Jungian analysis, I used to see the same therapist at the same time, on the same day, every week. Each week without fail, I would have what is called a 'big dream' the night before. This provided something to work with in the session next day. My inner world, my psyche, responded to this rhythm and helped me in the process. Interestingly, on the occasional times when I couldn't make my regular session, I still had the big dream. My inner world continued to propel me forward on my journey, even when my external circumstances were delaying my progress.

Jung believed that we have an innate instinct towards wholeness, and my own experiences have echoed that. Finding a rhythm is a way of dancing with this natural instinct. Regular practice, together with the right intention, commitment and dedication, create the transformational shifts needed to find freedom in our lives.

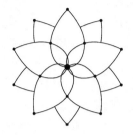

CHAPTER THIRTEEN

BEGINNING YOUR JOURNEY

It's now time to begin your journey into your chakras. Each of the seven sections that follow focus deeply on one of your seven chakras. As you read through these pages, you will gain an overall understanding of the nature of each chakra, how it interacts with and affects you, and why bringing it into balance is so important. In addition, you will find exercises and meditations to provide you with different ways of connecting with the chakra and bringing it into balance. Finally, at the end of each section, you will be prompted to dance the chakra that you've been focusing on, as a way of fully experiencing its power and blessings.

As you embark on your journey, I want you to know that you are not alone. I know that the journey within can feel isolating at times. Take heart in the knowledge that there are other brave souls who are also courageously taking this journey. In the words of the late mystic, Edgar Cayce: *Each soul enters with a mission. We all have a mission to perform.*

As you embark on your mission of finding and being your true self, remember to feel the collective support of other souls who are doing the same. As we each find freedom, flow and balance in our own life, so does that freedom, flow and balance ripple out into the world.

Let the journey begin ...

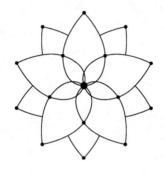

PART 3

MOVING YOUR
BASE CHAKRA

The first time I danced the base chakra it was very, very tribal. I was stamping my feet and shaking my hands. It was like I was part of a tribal ceremony. Ancestors surrounded me, and a circle of wise women. In the middle of the circle was a raging fire. It was strong and fierce, and I felt like I could manifest anything. Through this dance of the base chakra I learnt about survival—my own, through taking care of my body— and that to be physical is to be spiritual. The dance of the base chakra gave me an understanding of all those survival issues—especially my experience as a mother and my instinct to protect my child.

Jacki

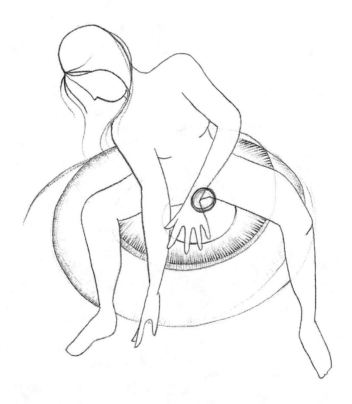

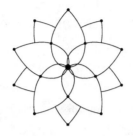

CHAPTER FOURTEEN

BODY WISDOM

Our journey begins at the base chakra, where we reconnect with the deep wisdom of our bodies. Our bodies remember all of our experiences. If our bodies could literally speak, there would be so many stories for them to tell. We could all write volumes of books on ourselves.

Our bodies remember the joyful experiences we have had in our lives—the exhilaration of the trampoline, the excitement of that first proper kiss—as well as less joyful times. Our bodies remember the feeling of being bullied at school, the sadness when our best friend moved away, the trauma of our dog dying, the death of our father, the grief of our divorce.

When deep feelings or traumas happen in our lives, we ideally experience the feelings at the time, assimilate them, and then discharge and release the energy. Think of how an animal behaves after it has had a fight or a scare. It experiences a high charge of energy and then literally shakes it off, releasing the trauma from its body.

Most of us humans have lost touch with this ancient instinctive release mechanism. Often, we don't fully accept or deal with our inner responses to intense or difficult experiences. Instead we suppress and block them. We try to avoid the pain or terror. We block the flow of energy and bury the memory and the feelings. The vibration of the trauma then becomes embedded into our bodies, woven into our muscles, our joints and our ligaments. Our blocked feelings of guilt, shame, pain and fear become the tensions in our bodies, the illnesses we don't understand.

The more we hold on to old feelings and traumas, the more restricted our bodies become. It can feel like we are wearing a coat of armour. For some people, you only have to look at their posture to see where they are holding on tightly to their pain. They may have sunken chests and hunched shoulders—you can practically see the pain they are carrying around in their hearts. Or they may stare down heavily at the floor, indicating a sadness that is making it difficult for them to hold their heads high.

When our bodies are restricted, it tends to be reflected in our lives in some way. If we can't physically let go of an old pain, we will find it challenging to let go in other areas of our lives, so our lives become restricted as well. For example, take the person with the sunken chest and hunched shoulders who is holding onto a pain in their heart. The longer that person carries the pain in their physical body, the more withdrawn and distanced they will become from others, so their relationships will suffer.

Conversely, when we find a way to release what we are holding in our bodies, a corresponding emotional release ripples out into our lives. When we find freedom of expression in our bodies, we find freedom in other aspects of our lives too.

Releasing blocked energy from our bodies is therefore vital for good health and overall wellbeing. We might work with therapists or healers, or do whatever inner work we are drawn to in order to understand and process our feelings and experiences, but to discharge the **holding** from our bodies is a vital (and often overlooked) step in the process.

In my Chakradance workshops, I have both experienced and witnessed the letting go of old energies from the body. There is often a release of emotion that takes place; and sometimes there is a memory, an image or a knowing that arises at the same time. As the old energy is discharged, our bodies feel more free, more fluid. It feels like an undoing of some kind. A space becomes cleared within our physical bodies and within our energy systems. Each time we release another trapped feeling from our bodies, we let go of an old pattern. We are freed up to be more present in the moment. We feel more alive.

We all have painful experiences from time to time; they are unavoidable parts of life. But what we don't need to do is carry the pain of those experiences in our bodies for the rest of our lives. As we connect with our base chakras, we tune into the wisdom of our bodies. When we tune into the wisdom of our bodies and let it guide us, we are able to release the energy that no longer serves us. We are able to find freedom in our bodies. We will then feel that freedom echo throughout our lives.

After dealing with some very painful back issues
this past week, I danced the base chakra. I had very
strong visions of a black panther perched on a rock
with teeth exposed. I wasn't afraid of the panther;
maybe I was the panther? As the dance continued,
I was a tribal woman singing and drumming. It
was a powerful dance and afterwards I almost
immediately experienced a significant release of much
of the pain I had been carrying in my lower back.

Mary

Time to try: *Releasing in the Moment*

When our base chakra is balanced, we are better able to prevent ourselves storing intense feelings and experiences in our bodies, rather than shaking them off. Perhaps you've just had an argument with your partner and you can feel the tightness in your chest. Or maybe your boss has made you angry and you notice that you are clenching your fists and tensing your whole body. It may even be something as simple as an encounter with a rude shop assistant that leads to tightness in your jaw. When we consciously notice our bodies holding onto energy that doesn't serve us, we can discharge it before it becomes too deeply embedded.

When you notice physical responses like these, that's your cue to do something to release the energy that is causing them. If you are at home and able to go to your sacred space, you can use the dance of the base chakra to immediately release the holding from your body. Begin by setting the intention of letting it go. Then, as you dance, tune into the experience and let the energy move through and out of your body.

If you are out and about or unable to dance, there are some simple movement exercises you can use in situations like these.

Find a place where you have some privacy and set the intention of discharging and releasing the feelings and experiences from your body. Then do one or both of the following exercises.

– SHAKING

Close your eyes and gently begin to shake up and down by bending and straightening your knees and shaking out your arms. Find your own rhythm and continue shaking for a few minutes. Use your breath and your intention to let go of feelings and energy you no longer need.

Stop and be still for a moment. Return to your normal breathing, and notice how you feel. You may want to do this a few times. As you do, keep noticing how you feel and how your body feels after each shake.

– SWEEPING

Begin by taking a few deep breaths. Next, brush your hands down your body using your fingertips to lightly sweep all the way from the top of your head down to your toes. Visualise the experience and the energy you are holding being swept away. Brush down the front of your body, then the back and the sides. Now repeat this movement but with your fingertips a few centimetres from your body, so you are sweeping your energy field. Keep sweeping down to the ground with the intention of letting go and releasing any unwanted energy.

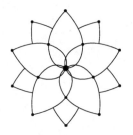

CHAPTER FIFTEEN

LETTING YOUR BODY do the TALKING

Dancing the base chakra plugs us into direct communication with our bodies. When we open ourselves up to hearing what our bodies have to say, our aches and pains can guide us to what is needed. As we move the base chakra, we breathe into our bodies and listen with heightened awareness. We become more conscious of the subtle body signals we are receiving as we dance.

Over time, you will learn to let your body be your wise guide. Perhaps you will find that your body is tired and needs to move gently on the floor. Or maybe your body will feel sluggish and you will feel called to shake it out. When was the last time you just stopped and tuned into your body, allowing it to whisper what it has to say to you? When was the last time you let your body do the talking?

One of my Chakradance participants, Imogen, woke up one morning feeling really sick. This was during the week when she was dancing (and focusing) on the base chakra. Normally in this situation, she would take some medication and hope she would feel better. Instead, she felt called to listen to her body. She felt as though she wanted some camomile tea, and her husband kindly made it for her. She took one sip and rejected it immediately, as it made her feel worse.

Even though Imogen was feeling dreadful, she recognised that she felt a deep connection to her body. It was as though she could hear and understand it, like she never had before. In particular, she noticed that her sense of smell was heightened. She then started to sense which herbs from her garden her body needed and she asked her husband to pick the leaves for her. She sniffed the leaves and, in spite of the awful smell, she knew that the herbs were exactly what she needed to feel better.

Imogen had never before had knowledge of herbs and tea, so this was all new for her. In that moment, she completely understood how animals in nature know what they need and how to cure themselves. She felt like an animal herself. She knew the exact proportions for the tea and how best to drink it. Within an hour she felt completely back to normal, with no sign of sickness. This deep connection with her body felt like a new-found gift to her.

Symptoms as signals

Our bodies are vast, often untapped sources of wisdom. They are constantly communicating with us and telling us what they need. They communicate through our physical symptoms. A symptom is a sign—a bright, flashing signal that something is wrong. Often we focus on trying to get rid of the symptom by taking medication to numb the pain or mitigate the effect, so we can get on with our lives. But chances are the symptom will keep coming back, and quite possibly get even stronger, until we learn to act on what the symptom is trying to communicate to us.

Imagine you are driving your car, when a warning light starts to flash on your dashboard. The light is a signal to alert you to the fact that your car is running low on oil, gas or brake fluid. When this happens, we don't try to stop the light from flashing at us. We listen to what it has to say and we take action. Our physical symptoms are just like the flashing lights on our cars. We need to listen to the messages our bodies are sending us, then take the actions needed to heal.

I would always recommend a visit to the doctor to find out more about any symptom that arises and gain appropriate medical advice. But in conjunction with that, I encourage you to tune in to your body. An important part of the journey towards good health is building a relationship with our bodies, where we establish a form of communication and a level of respect. We need to learn the language of the body and how to interpret its signals. These will be different for each of us. But the more we connect with our bodies and listen to them, the deeper our understanding of the signals will be.

Begin by taking notice if your back, neck or any other part of you starts hurting, then ask yourself questions. Does this happen when you feel you are not getting the support you need? What happens to your body when you are challenged or when you are criticised? When you feel tense, where does your body tense up? What is happening in your life when you get a sore throat? A skin rash? To understand the wisdom of our bodies, we need to start paying greater attention to physical symptoms. If we keep ignoring the messages, they tend to get louder and louder until we are forced to stop and pay attention.

There is a great deal of research showing the interconnectedness of mind and body. They are not separate from each other. An intricate web connects the two. Just think about how we blush when we are embarrassed, or get sweaty palms and a racing heart when we feel nervous. Just imagine for a moment what loneliness, heartbreak and anger could do to our bodies, if ignored and left to grow unchecked over time.

I didn't realise how much my body needed to move and then, yes! It felt afterwards like it needed to retreat. The interesting feelings were around acknowledging how primal my body wanted to get and how stagnant and constricted she had felt before the dance.

Dana

Time to try: *Listening as Your Body Speaks*

I have found this simple exercise to be incredibly revealing. All it requires is for you to write out how your symptoms feel. This can give you clues as to what your underlying emotional and psychological states may be. It is literally like giving our body the opportunity to speak.

For example, if you have a headache, describe how the pain feels. Really get into it and write down everything you can about it. Maybe it feels pounding, intense, hot, restrictive, thumping, blinding, overwhelming or tight. Describe it as vividly as you can.

Next, think about what's happening in your life right now. Could your description of your headache also apply to any other parts of your life? Remember, this headache has a message for you. There is a reason you are experiencing it. Something in your life needs to change.

To give another example, maybe you have a sore foot. How does this pain feel? Is it restrictive? Does it hurt to move forward? Is it stopping you in your tracks? Where else in your life are similar feelings occurring? What's the message that you need to hear?

If you are struggling to describe how your pain feels, write down whether your symptom has a temperature or a colour.

Describe any images that come to mind as you focus on it. You may want to draw the pain or paint it. It doesn't matter so much what method you use, as long as it helps you to build a relationship with your body and learn how to communicate with it. Keep asking questions and looking to see where similar feelings are at play in your life. Once you can see an issue, then you can begin to do something about it. If we keep numbing ourselves to our symptoms, the voices of our bodies go unheard.

I once had a sinus infection and I kept finding myself saying, 'I can't breathe.' When I tuned in further, I realised that there was an aspect of my life that energetically made me feel like I couldn't breathe. As soon as I became conscious of this, I did what I could to clear the sinus infection, but I also took steps to make changes to the 'unbreathable' situation in my life.

The next time I got a sinus infection, I immediately looked for a situation in my life that could be related to it. I saw that I was working way too much and had not been giving myself any space or downtime. As soon as I realised this, I took a walk along the beach and scheduled in some time with my girlfriends. My sinus infection cleared up very quickly after that.

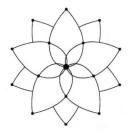

CHAPTER SIXTEEN

RECONNECTING to YOUR BODY

Our experiences in the modern world can leave us feeling disconnected from our bodies, which creates a whole host of problems for us. Our bodies are our homes, our temples, our lovers for this lifetime. When we become disconnected from them, we can become like the walking dead—homeless, lost and empty.

Many years ago, I discovered the work of an amazing Jungian analyst and author named Marion Woodman. She described the condition of being disconnected from our bodies perfectly: *Matter without spirit is a corpse. Spirit without matter is a ghost.* Just take a moment to reflect on that powerful statement. Before we can do any of the wonderful things we plan to do with our lives, we must first come fully home to our bodies.

Sadly, we live in a culture that often promotes a ghost-like existence. Many of us spend so much time thinking, analysing and worrying about things that our energy gets constantly sent upwards to our heads. We literally put 'mind over matter' so much of the time. Many of us are also so busy with our jobs, families and to-do lists that our energy gets stretched in lots of different directions. When this happens, we are left feeling energetically scattered by the end of the day.

One of the main functions of the base chakra is to help us become grounded. You may have come across the term 'grounding' before, but what does it actually mean?

When we are grounded, we are energetically connected to, and fully present in, our bodies. I know when I am grounded: my breath deepens, everything seems to slow down a little, and I become more in tune with my physical senses. I become more present in the here and now.

Making time each day to ground yourself can really make a big difference to how you deal with daily life. If a challenging situation comes your way at work, you will be able to stand firm without flying off the handle or feeling overwhelmed. If a difficult family situation arises, you will be able to stay present and calm and not get swept away with the emotions that may arise in you.

We often become 'ungrounded' when we have difficult decisions to make, as we can get lost in a barrage of thoughts. However, this is an especially important time for us to ground, as it will help us to become more focused.

Dancing the base chakra is one of the most powerful and enjoyable ways of grounding that I know. The music of the base chakra helps to draw our energy back into our bodies. The tribal beats call us to move our legs and feet and connect us with the earth. Our dance helps us to calm the chaos, and become more connected and present.

A Chakradance participant, Kirsten, has always felt unsafe in this world. Although she feels like she has a tribe, she's never felt truly at home. When she began dancing the base chakra, she felt uncomfortable at first and was crying. She then had a powerful vision of a white buffalo. As she danced with this vision, she felt herself sink, surrender and become supported by Mother Earth. She suddenly realised that her feet were feeling the carpet and ground beneath her, in a way they never had before. This was a profound experience for Kirsten, as she felt she had come home to her body. She now calls on white buffalo to help her whenever she feels she needs grounding.

Time to try: *Grounding Techniques*

In addition to dancing your base chakra, there are some easy ways that you can become more grounded in your day-to-day life. Anything that deepens your connection with your physical body will help you ground, so things like physical exercise or having a massage are great ways to stay grounded on a regular basis. Over the years I have discovered other techniques as well, which I share below. I encourage you to try them out and feel which ones work best for you. I encourage you to also take notice of the things you are already doing naturally to ground, and consciously use these when you need to.

– SPEND TIME IN NATURE

A simple way of grounding is to spend more time in nature. When was the last time you walked barefoot on the earth or just sat quietly in a park? Remember the feeling it gave you? When we connect with the earth, we anchor our energy and plug ourselves into the richness that Mother Earth has to offer. We can literally ground out our stresses, worries or overwhelming feelings by allowing Mother Earth to absorb them from us. It helps to think of the earth as an enormous, loving mother. Just as a small child runs to her mother for comfort when she feels scared or hurt, so too we can turn to Mother Earth. When a mother hugs her child, she takes away the child's pain and transforms it with love. This is what the great mother can do for all of us.

– MINDFUL WALKING

Set the intention to walk mindfully through your day. I once did a meditation retreat where we did mindful walking for hours at a time over many days. Obviously, walking at a meditation retreat is quite different from walking around the supermarket, but we can be mindfully present anywhere. As you walk out of your home each morning, set the intention of walking consciously. Feel your feet on the ground below you, smell the air as you breathe, listen to the sounds around you. Walk through your day with your mind attuned to what you are actually doing, right now, in each moment. Feel yourself fully present in your body.

– TUNE INTO YOUR SENSES

I was introduced to this exercise by my Jungian therapist, Sally. It is extremely simple and yet very powerful. It can be used any time you want to ground your energy in your body, but is particularly useful if you have disconnected from your body through some kind of shock, extreme fear or overwhelming emotion.

Close your eyes and take three deep breaths. Name five sounds you can hear. Then gently open your eyes and name five things you can see.

If you still feel disconnected, use your other senses to deepen the connection. Smell some different aromatherapy oils, taste some different flavours, or touch some different fabrics and be aware of the sensations. Engaging fully with our senses leads us home to our bodies and to the now.

During the base Chakradance yesterday, I kept seeing images of this wolf, surrounded by amazing red light. I felt as if I was the wolf, scratching and crawling my way out in order to survive and be free. I was so dizzy after and felt almost motion sick. I thought at one point that I was going to be sick. The last three years for me have been the most challenging of my life. I went through a divorce and now am a single mother of a three year old. I left my home of twenty years to be close to my family. I am the primary provider for me and my daughter. And this dance felt as if I were crawling out of the darkness and into the light. The wolf and I were one—wild and free.

Shannie

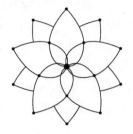

CHAPTER SEVENTEEN

RECONNECTING to YOUR INSTINCTS

In addition to helping us reconnect to the wisdom of our bodies, the base chakra calls us to reconnect to our deep inner instincts. We are part of the animal species and yet, in our efforts to become civilised, we have lost a lot of the amazing gifts that are natural to us by allowing them to become buried. Obviously, it would not be desirable for us to completely revert to wild animal status! But we can relearn how to draw on our animal instincts, to help guide us and keep us safe in life.

Have you ever felt a ripple of fear travel up your spine? That's your instincts giving you a clear message that there is some form of danger nearby. When we sense danger, our fight or flight mechanism automatically kicks in. But if we are disconnected from our bodies, we might not recognise the threat.

When we bury our instincts in the unconscious, our fears become distorted; it's as if they become disconnected from real time. We either don't pick up on the danger or become para-lysed by fear when there is no danger present. When we are in tune with our bodies and our instincts, the ripple of fear acts as a guide to give us a genuine, timely warning. When we learn to trust this physical signal, fear becomes our friend.

We no longer live in caves, dependent on hunting and gathering for our dinner while on the lookout for wild beasts. Our world has changed, we have changed, and yet we still need to survive. We need to put food on the table, support ourselves and our families, and do what we can to stay safe and well. We still need our instincts for survival. So we need to tune into this part of us that gives us timely warnings. Just as we need to reconnect with our bodies, we need to release the reins on the animal within us.

The dance of the base chakra does just that. It connects us directly back to our instinctive animal nature.

We can further enhance the connection with our animal instincts by opening ourselves up to the wisdom that animals can teach us. In shamanic cultures, it is believed that we all have power or spirit animals. Each animal carries its own wisdom and power and, when we become attuned to these animals, it is as though we take on their unique powers. A dolphin, for example, may guide you to play more, find the positive in things, or do things that help you feel joyful. An encounter with a deer may guide you to bring more gentleness and grace into your life.

Dancing the base chakra is a powerful way to connect with these spirit animals and receive the guidance they have for us. One of my Chakradance participants, Mallory, had a jaguar appear as she danced. She was raised in rough circumstances and didn't always have the highest moral code. She did what she could to survive when she was younger. However, since getting married and having children, she has lived life with integrity in everything she does. For Mallory, the jaguar was validation. Jaguars represent virtue, honour and trustworthiness, and she feels the jaguar came forward in her dance to reinforce her evolution and spiritual journey.

I've found that different animals come to me at different times of my life. And they always appear at a time when their specific power is needed.

A few years ago, I was going through one of the most challenging times that I have ever experienced. When I reached a point of feeling overwhelmed and probably more scared than I have ever been in my life, a tiger appeared in my dance. At first I could only feel his presence while I danced, but gradually I could feel his energy next to me as I moved through my day. I remember one particular day very clearly. I was walking down a busy street, feeling my tiger prowling low next to me. I remember thinking, 'Am I making this up?' Just then, a truck passed with a big tiger logo painted on its side. Then a car went past with a tiger sticker on the back. A few minutes later, I walked into a newsagency and saw a tiger on the front cover of a magazine on the counter. I had to laugh at all the confirmations I was being given.

As I continued to dance with tiger energy in my Chakradance practice, I received the gift he was there to give me. He was teaching me how to face issues head on. He was showing me that I needed to face my deepest fears and tackle them directly. There was no point in hoping they would go away or trying to find an easy way out. I needed to step fully into my own power and strength, something I had never really done before. Looking back, I feel my tiger spirit both protected me and imbued me with the courage I couldn't quite find on my own. He was by my side as I travelled through the dark passage that I needed to take.

Calling on your spirit animal

As you move your base chakra, you may connect with a spirit animal that could be helpful in your life at this moment. You may feel it as an energetic presence, see its image, or just have a knowingness.

When we first meet our animal, it can take some time to recognise and understand the gift it is there to give us, the lesson it is there to teach us. There is a lot of information available on the symbolic meanings of different animal spirits. This can be a great place to start to learn more about the possible gifts your animal has come to share with you.

I have found that the most powerful way to build a connection is to dance with the energy of your animal. When we invite the animal spirit into our energy field, it's like a merging. The spirit of your animal is moving through your energy field and you are moving through the animal's energy. It's not just dancing; we move as though we **are** our animal. This helps us to feel the animal's energy more deeply, to embody its qualities, and to understand its message for us.

After you dance, keep tuning into your animal and stay open to any messages it may have for you. This type of work can be subtle. But in my experience it is always deeply powerful, if you trust it. As you step back into your daily life, have the intention of seeing your life through the eyes of your animal. Ask yourself how your animal would respond to certain situations. How would it deal with the people you are encountering in your life? What is it there to show you?

Meditation: *Meeting Your Spirit Animal*

Try the following guided meditation as a way of connecting with a spirit animal. It can be helpful to do this meditation before you dance; or you may choose to do it regularly, to connect with different animals. You are likely to encounter different animals at different times, depending on what is needed in your life at that moment.

You can do this meditation by reading the following steps, pausing after each one to imagine what has been described, or by listening to it with my voice-over guidance on the Base Meditation: Meeting Your Spirit Animal track: [refer to page vi]

1. Prepare your sacred space and yourself. Softly close your eyes and take three slow, deep breaths.

2. Imagine you are sitting in a beautiful field, filled with brightly-coloured flowers. Your back is resting against a big old tree. In the distance you can see a pathway leading down into a deep valley. You feel drawn to walk towards it.

3. As you step onto the path, you notice an animal standing guard at the edge. You feel safe with this animal. It begins to walk beside you, as you travel deeper down the path. This animal feels like your guardian and is here to ensure you have a safe journey in this meditation.

4. As you continue down the path, the overhanging branches become thicker, and you feel as though you are walking through a tunnel made of trees. Although it's dark, sunlight dapples through, lighting your way.

5. You find yourself standing at the entrance to a cave. There are large crystals on either side of the entrance, creating a sacred gateway. You feel drawn inside the cave. A small light glows in a lantern at the back of the cave, and you know that it has been lit especially for you. Near the light, you see that there are steps leading down into another cave deep in the earth. You can sense a presence down in the cave and you know that this is an animal, your power animal, waiting to meet you.

6. As you slowly move down the steps, you see glowing eyes in the darkness. These are the eyes of an animal. They are gentle and caring. You recognise these eyes; they feel familiar to you. As your eyes adjust to the darkness, a face begins

to form around the eyes and then a whole body is visible to you. Your power animal stands before you.

7. Sit with your animal and receive what it has to offer you. It may circle you, sit with you or speak to you. It may have something to show you. It may have a gift of some kind for you. Spend this time simply being with your animal guide.

8. It is now time to return to your daily life. Thank your animal. Know that you can return to visit your animal whenever you please.

9. You make your way back up the stairs. The glow of the lantern lights your way out of the cave. You pass through the sacred gateway of crystals and begin to walk back through the tunnel of trees. You notice that your guardian animal is still with you.

10. You travel all the way back up the pathway until you return to the field. You thank your guardian animal, and you walk alone across the field and back to the big old tree. You sit and rest with your back against the tree and look at the brightly-coloured flowers.

11. Take three deep breaths and slowly open your eyes.

If you struggle to see or feel an animal during your meditation, please don't worry. What tends to happen is that your animal will appear to you in some other way during the coming days. You might dream of an animal or a real live animal may enter your life in a significant way. Trust your animal is there and will make contact with you in a way that you can recognise.

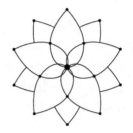

CHAPTER EIGHTEEN

CONNECTING WITH YOUR ANCESTORS

The base chakra is also known as the root chakra. Not only does this chakra help keep us rooted to the earth, it also connects us to our ancestral roots, our roots of origin. It is the energetic connection to our bloodline.

We not only carry the genes of our ancestors, we also carry a cellular and energetic imprint of them. Everything from their beliefs and their patterns to their unresolved issues can be passed down to us. Just reflect for a moment on your parents, your grandparents, your great-grandparents. You can probably see some physical resemblances, but can you also see some character traits, spiritual beliefs or behaviours that were passed down the family line? There will be some wonderful energetic DNA that you have been blessed with, but for most of us there will also be some unresolved patterns or outdated beliefs that need healing.

You may be able to tell from your family history that you have a disposition toward certain things. Perhaps there has been a lot of creative or musical ability throughout your family? You may have come from a lineage of great sporting ability or intuitive psychics. You may, at the same time, come from a family that has battled alcoholism, mental illness, or had severe issues around money or poverty. We may not necessarily inherit every trait, but looking back at our family history can show us some of the issues we may want to look out for, the things we may be more prone to.

Our energetic inheritance is quite often unconscious, and we don't always see how our ancestral patterns are impacting on our day-to-day lives. Our energetic genes can affect our present day relationships and our bodies. They can even influence our choice of career and partners. One of the most healing aspects of dancing the base chakra is to bring these patterns into consciousness. We can embody the wisdom that our ancestors have for us, and we can release and heal our ancient wounds.

Sarah had a slow start to her dance. As she began to move, all she could hear was her mother telling her as a child to stop showing off. But she didn't let the voice stop her. Instead she knew instinctively that it was coming up in order to be dealt with. After all, Sarah didn't believe she was a show-off. That was a judgement passed down to her by her mother. Through the dance, she was able to let go of the energy around that judgement and find a new sense of freedom in her life.

Our ancestral energy can also travel back many generations. When Patty danced, she was taken back to her Italian ancestral lineage. During the dance she heard the anguish of women suffering and crying, while being burnt for using their magic and intuition. She could feel the guilt and the punishment rippling down the generations. She could also see why there was so much suffering among the women on the Italian side of her family. They had lost their gypsy souls. They had lost their voices. And when that happened, they turned instead to alcohol and antidepressants.

Patty was determined to stop this ancestral pattern. As she danced, she felt a bright light encircling her whole body. She saw that she was here to protect and heal the past, by reigniting the spirit of her lost Italian gypsy heritage. She had a moment of release, which she described as being like an exorcism. Her body got so hot that she started to shake. She received a message to 'protect the sacred.' Her dance ended with a community of women holding hands, with the intention of protecting that which was sacred to them.

Healing a family pattern is much like healing a physical wound. Once it is healed, it leaves us. We can literally move these patterns out of our bodies and release them from our energy fields, so they no longer steer the direction of our lives. We can make new choices, find a new way of being. In many ways, it's as if we can begin writing a new story for ourselves and our families. When we release energetic wounds, they are released from the past, the present and the future. When we heal ourselves, we are not only clearing space in our own lives, we are clearing the energetic debris from the lives of our ancestors and our future generations.

Sometimes when we heal our energy, others will feel it. When Brianna danced the base chakra, she had an experience that involved seeing and releasing a pattern from her mother's side of the family. As she was dancing, her mother phoned her because she could feel something was going on and wanted to check that Brianna was okay. Energetic healing is like electricity. We can't see it, but its effects are deeply powerful.

As you move your base chakra, you may experience the wonderful feelings our families can bring us, such as a sense of comfort, support and belonging. You may connect more deeply with the wisdom and the positive traits that have been bestowed upon you by your ancestors. Or you may receive a memory, an insight, a vision of something that needs healing. Deep feelings may surface, and your body may move in a way that lets them go.

As with your power animal, more insight may come after your dance. You may have a dream or a memory, or you may even find yourself being contacted by a family member. Just stay open and aware and hold a willingness for healing.

> *This morning, as I danced the base chakra, I found myself connected to my Native American ancestors. I have Lakota blood (albeit way back and mostly unacknowledged by anyone in my family until I was thirty years old—I'm sixty-five now). I embodied an older male chieftain. I was alone, drawing in the wise ones. I felt very rooted, very ceremonial like, and honoured by the visit from my ancestors.*
>
> Jill

Time to try: *Ancestral Healing*

You may choose to spend some time diving deeper into your ancestral history, with the intention of releasing any negative patterns that are being passed down through the generations. The more conscious we can become of these patterns, the more we can take steps to change them.

On a practical level, you may choose to trace your family tree and look for any recurring patterns being passed down. You may want to talk to members of your family to find out as much information as you can.

On an energetic level, you may try the following exercise for releasing negative energetic patterns in your ancestral history:

1. While sitting in your sacred space, close your eyes and imagine that your parents are sitting behind you. Take a few minutes to feel their energy. Even if you have never met your parents, you can still call them in, as it is their energy you are connecting with. You may ask them to show you any patterns that need healing. Even if nothing comes to you, know that you are setting an intention for healing and releasing any family patterns that are not serving you. You are choosing to end any negative cycles.

2. Now imagine your grandparents sitting behind your parents. And then your great-grandparents behind them, and so on. Take a few minutes to feel the energy of your ancestors behind you.

3. As you tune into your ancestral line, imagine seeing any negative patterns you have inherited as energetic cords connecting you to your family. You may see or feel these cords as ropes, chains or whatever vision comes to you. They may feel like thick or thin threads. Spend some time sensing these energetic cords.

4. Now visualise cutting these cords and releasing the negative patterns that are attached to them. To cut the cords, you may choose to use a golden sword or scissors. Or you may choose to simply unplug the cords from you. Whatever visualisation you use, ensure that you have fully cut the ties. As you release the cords, imagine them dissolving, freeing you and also your ancestors from the negative patterns.

5. To complete this exercise, take a few minutes to focus on your breathing and reflect on how you feel. You may want to journal about your experience and write down any feelings or visions that came to you during the exercise.

You may feel the need to repeat this exercise several times. Each time, tune in and see if you can sense any remaining cords. They may feel weaker or they may have been fully released. If needed, repeat this exercise until you feel the cords have fully dissolved. I feel our ancestors are calling us to do this healing work, not only to heal them, but so that we can heal ourselves as well as our future generations.

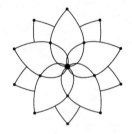

CHAPTER NINETEEN

DANCING the BASE CHAKRA

*I believe I have found my life's purpose here in the base
chakra. I was having a hard time connecting to what
it is I'm supposed to be doing before dancing the base
chakra, and now it is so clear to me. It has really helped
me to integrate the spiritual into the physical world.*

Caley

It is now time to move your base chakra. Create your sacred
space and prepare yourself for the dance, as outlined in Part 2:
Preparing for Your Journey. Once you are ready, begin by taking
three slow, deep breaths and planting your feet firmly on the
ground. Imagine the soles of your feet energetically opening, and
visualise them beginning to grow roots like a tree—roots that
push down through the layers of the soil, right to the heart of
the planet's crystalline core. Breathe in through your body and

out down through your roots as they merge with the layers of the earth.

When you are ready, play the Move Your Base Chakra music [refer to page vi] and feel the vibration of the crystal bowl pulsing at the base of your spine. Close your eyes and surrender to the pulsating, earthy beats.

The dance of the base chakra is a raw, primal dance. As you give yourself permission to truly surrender into your primal self, you will find your body begin to move in its own unique way. You may feel drawn to move on all fours or get low to the ground. As you come out of your head and anchor into your body, you will find yourself being moved by your wild, instinctive energy. You may find yourself emphasising movements of your legs and feet, as you anchor your energy down and connect with Mother Earth.

Once you have finished your dance, take three slow, deep breaths, then sit down to create your mandala art. Refer to page 24 for directions on how to do this.

Chanting the base chakra

Each chakra has a specific mantra sound. When chanted, this sound helps to activate the chakra. I will talk about this in more detail in the throat chakra section (Chapter 44: Sacred Singing and Chanting). The mantra sound for the base chakra is LAM (pronounced as LUM). You might like to take a few minutes to practise chanting this sound.

Sit peacefully and bring your awareness to your breathing. Inhale fully through your nose. As you exhale, vocalise the mantra LAM while focusing your awareness at your perineum area. I recommend chanting for around five minutes.

Take notice of any feelings, memories, images or sensations that come up for you as you chant. Spend a few minutes coming back to your natural breathing to finish.

Base chakra affirmation:
I love every part of my body.
Every cell is filled with energy and vitality.

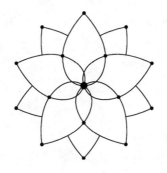

PART 4

MOVING YOUR
SACRAL CHAKRA

As soon as I started dancing the sacral chakra, the most magical things started happening. I felt so much more sensual and feminine. My husband started noticing the changes and his attitude started changing.

Our relationship improved so much. There was just an energy in the house and I can't explain it, but I felt like a teenager experiencing her first thoughts and feelings of sexuality and sensuality.

Nadine

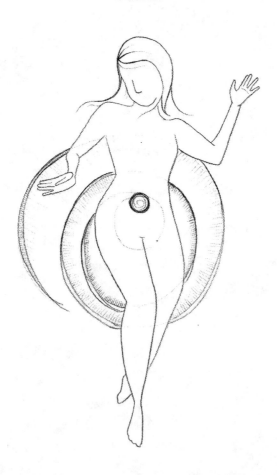

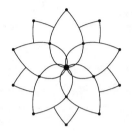

CHAPTER TWENTY

the SACRED FEMININE

The next step on our journey is to move our sacral chakra and feel the wisdom of the sacred feminine. The sacred feminine is an energy that we all, whether female or male, have within us. We need to embrace it, if we are to be truly in touch with our feelings, our sensuality and our passion.

Many of us have grown up with some fixed ideas about what it means to be feminine. We learn from our families, our friends, our cultures and our experiences that we should behave in a certain way, look a certain way, dress a certain way, and so on. Many of us have unconsciously created masks that we feel we must wear, in order to be accepted and loved.

However, true feminine energy is a life force within, which is not confined by what we wear, how we speak, or the kind of job we do. The sacred feminine is sensual, life-giving, intuitive, tender and wild. If we are to live a passionate and creative life, we need to learn to pull off our masks and own this part of ourselves with honour, dignity and grace. We need her, and the world needs her.

Our feminine energy is not something that we need to study. We won't find her in a book or by searching outside of ourselves. To reclaim this wisdom, we need to travel within and remember who we are by nature. We need to peel back the layers within ourselves and shine a light on her. She is there, just waiting to be revealed.

Dancing the sacral chakra is like opening a doorway which leads directly to this wisdom. When we surrender into the sensual, tantalising, passionate music, we meet all the embodiments of the sacred feminine within us. We dance our softness, our darkness, our wildness and our grace.

Last year, a friend and I attended an event that was all about discovering and celebrating the feminine. As part of the event, we were asked to complete a quiz to discover how in touch we were with our femininity. The questions included things like: 'Do you like wearing sexy lingerie?' and 'Do you like having manicures and facials?' As we sat with this quiz, I noticed that my friend looked as if she were about to explode. She whispered loudly to me that she was going to fail the feminine quiz, because she hated nail polish and facials. In fact, she felt most feminine when she had dirt under her fingernails from digging in the garden or when firing an arrow during her archery class.

The sacred feminine is most alive within us when we are being true to who we are. The feminine can be pretty and delicate, but she can also be untamed, dark and fierce. When we truly allow the power of the feminine into our lives, we discover our own beauty. It doesn't matter what clothes (or lingerie) we are wearing; it's about how we wear our soul. It doesn't matter how old we are; we can embrace the beauty and wisdom of every year we are privileged enough to have lived.

We embrace the sacred feminine when we follow our inner voice over the voices of others. We don't need to be confined by whatever we were taught about femininity. When we take off those masks, that's when we begin to truly live. We belly laugh. We follow our dreams with wild abandon. We fiercely protect those we love. We nurture and we graciously receive. We have an aliveness pulsing through our bodies. The sacred feminine is already within you; she is within each and every one of us.

The sacred feminine needs nurturing to keep her fully present and awake in our lives. If we don't feed ourselves with creativity, passion and wildness, we can become disconnected from her. We can start to feel flat, barren or dried out. Our lives can feel monotonous and dull, as though we are just going through the motions. Our bodies can begin to feel stiff and rigid.

The dance of the sacral chakra is like a sacred ritual, a ceremony in honour of her.

When Tracy danced the sacral chakra, she found herself softly saying, 'Welcome back, wild woman.' She also received the message to find more time for pleasure in her life. As she moved, she felt the wild and dark parts of herself dancing with soft love and light. The physical pain she had been holding in her groin and hip dissolved and she began to cry. Not a sad cry, but a thankful and releasing cry, knowing that she would not deprive herself of pleasure any longer.

The more we nurture the sacred feminine, the more we are able to hear her voice. She calls to us to dance more, play more, get outside and be wild. She guides us to follow that creative impulse and live that dream. When we dance in harmony with the sacred feminine, our creativity blossoms, our relationships deepen, and we feel alive and excited about our lives.

*When I danced the sacral dance, the feminine dance, one that I have done many times before, I was overwhelmed with the **power** of the feminine. Before, perhaps, it has seemed soft and gentle, but now I really felt its wild, fierce-mother, protective, powerful energy. I had visions of wild mountain lions protecting their fluffy babies with claws, roars and teeth. It came when I needed such energy in my life.*

Suzanne

As I met the sacred feminine in my dance, I had a real sense of what this energy feels like when she is healed, whole and balanced. I felt regal, powerful, sensual and sexual—but free from the need for an 'other' to validate that.

Beth Ann

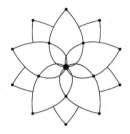

CHAPTER TWENTY-ONE

FEELING HER THROUGH PASSION

We can find the sacred feminine through passion. Passion is her food, her sustenance. It feeds this part of us emotionally, energetically and even on a cellular level. To find the sacred feminine within, ask yourself: What lights me up? What floods me with energy, vitality and radiance? That's what we all need to find.

Passion is like an elixir for our body and soul, but it's important to understand what true passion is. Passion is different from chasing a high. It's not about gambling, wild shopping sprees, or whatever else helps us escape from life. These things may give us an initial surge of energy, but ultimately they disconnect us from ourselves. True, healthy passion deepens our connection with ourselves. It has a unique quality to it, like liquid gold flowing through our bodies. It helps us feel more present, awake and alive. It connects us with the sacred feminine.

It's easy to think that our passion is fuelled by others, especially in a romantic way. To an extent, this is true. But if we only connect with passion through another, and they leave us, then our passion goes too. We are left feeling empty and craving this energy. That can cause us to search for it in all the wrong places. So we need to be able to feed and nurture ourselves first.

One of my personal passions is dance. It has been an ongoing part of my life, sometimes more prominent than at other times, but always calling me. I know now that whenever I give myself the gift of truly surrendering into my own dance, especially through Chakradance, my passion is fully reignited. It is a way for me to plug straight into a source of magical, vibrant energy. Whenever I dance, I feel this way. If I stop giving myself time to dance, I begin to feel depleted in some way. I now know that I need to dance regularly. Dance is my connection to the wild feminine.

Many of us need to learn to value the role passion plays in our lives. You may have a secret love of playing an instrument, writing poetry, or swimming in the ocean. But perhaps you have cast this love aside, considering it a waste of time, not important, or something that couldn't possibly be taken seriously by others. Perhaps you have buried your passion so deeply, you don't even know what lights you up anymore?

Whether you have buried your passion or cast it aside, chances are that somewhere along the way, you internalised a message that passion was not needed, deserved or rewarded. You have disowned this part of you. It's time to get it back.

Time to try: *Reignite Your Passion*

If you know what lights you up, make a commitment to spend more time doing whatever that is. If you have buried your passion, it's time to reignite it.

I have found that the things that activate our passion are often the things we were naturally drawn to as children. What made you feel playful and joyous as a child? If you are struggling to find your passion, I recommend spending some time reflecting on your life and writing down anything you can think of that you loved doing as a child. It's not necessarily about searching out there for new things that might light you up; it's about remembering what passions have been with you all along.

Even if something you loved as a child doesn't make sense in your adult life, maybe you can find a new version of it. Reflect on the following questions and notice any themes or memories that help you remember your passion:

- What have you always loved doing?
- What interests did you have as a child?
- What games did you play?
- What were you naturally good at?
- What were you doing when you last felt a flood of joy move through you?
- When do you feel most alive? When connecting with other people? Travelling? Doing something creative?
- What makes you shine from the inside out?
- What section of the bookstore are you drawn to?
- What did you want to be when you grew up?

Passion is already inside you. This is about removing the layers that are covering it up and letting its vibrancy move through you.

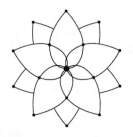

CHAPTER TWENTY-TWO

LIVING the RHYTHMS of the FEMININE

Many of us have forgotten how to live the rhythms of the feminine. When we invite her back into our lives, we open ourselves up to remembering ancient wisdom. We reconnect with sacred mysteries and knowledge.

In Egypt, there is an ancient temple dedicated to the Goddess Hathor. Hathor personifies the principles of the sacred feminine, sexuality, and the arts—dancing, music, sculpture and so on. Her temple, believed to be over 4,000 years old, is where sacred initiations by priestesses took place, and where sacred knowledge was taught. The temple has many buildings within, each one dedicated to a specific purpose, eg. birthing and the tantric arts. Carved into the walls of this grand sandstone temple is information about astrology, astronomy and alchemy. People who visit the temple claim to feel the presence of feminine, sweet, gentle energy.

What struck me most about hearing about the Temple of Hathor is how revered and sacred the feminine once was. Sadly, it has become lost and distorted over the thousands of years since this temple was built. It seems to me that it is time for the sacred feminine to rise again. It is time for us all to feel her gentle power, wisdom and mystery within us.

As women, we can feel her presence in our bodies as we experience the natural rhythm of our monthly cycle. Many of us have come to dread this time of the month and do all we can to pretend it's not happening. But as our uterus sheds its lining, just as a snake sheds its skin, we are at one with nature. It is as though each month we are physically cleansed and emotionally replenished, ready to begin with the next cycle. Shifting our perspective on our monthly cycle will deepen our connection with the sacred feminine.

As I write this book, I am moving into the season of menopause. I can feel that I am transitioning into a new rhythm of the feminine. I'm experiencing all of the typical physical and emotional signs of menopause, and my initial reactions were fear, loss and sadness.

When I recently danced the sacral chakra, an image of Kali, the great Hindu goddess, appeared. Kali is frightening to look at and is often described as the death goddess. Dancing with her was a new experience for me, and I felt all I could do was fully surrender myself to her dance and be open to what she had to bring me.

For me, the most surprising part of this new rhythm so far is my increased surge in creativity. Kali is the embodiment of Mother Nature. She cleanses away the old with natural storms and fires, to make the ground fertile for new crops and life. It feels like the end of my personal fertility is opening me up to a whole new creative way of being. Instead of birthing babies, I'm giving birth to all the ideas that are arising within me. As

I danced the sacral chakra today, I felt like a dancing goddess with many arms. Each hand was cupped like a womb, holding and incubating a creative idea. I'm now feeling excited about this new feminine rhythm I'm dancing in.

The cycle of our bodies connects us to the greater rhythms of nature. We live the cycles of the moon, the changing of the seasons, the dance of maiden, mother and crone. The mystery of the sacred feminine is right here within us.

I have a small circle of friends who try to get together every full moon, so we can engage in various rituals to connect with the sacred feminine. We have walked through national parks, dived into fairy pools, danced around fires and thrown stones into the ocean, with the intention of releasing what we no longer need. These are no ordinary girls' nights out. Although we laugh, often cry, and share stories, dreams and fears, there is something deeper going on. We choose the full moon, not because we are hippies, but because there is a cycle to what we do, a rhythm. The full moon is symbolic of the wild feminine, and that is what we are connecting with, together and within ourselves.

Something deeply magical always happens on these nights. It often feels like we are entering into a different time, a different realm. It feels like we are connecting with the priestesses of the past and opening up to a wisdom that we can't normally access. The atmosphere feels both wild and sacred. There is a certain mystery that we tap into, when we invoke the sacred feminine.

What's amazing is that, after these nights, we all typically notice a shift of some kind within ourselves or in our daily lives. Something that has been blocked moves. Something that didn't make sense now does. We have learnt that ritual, intention and feminine magic are incredibly powerful and highly sacred.

Whether you are male or female, reflect on some ways in which you can embrace the rhythms of the sacred feminine in your life. This may mean finding time one night each week for a relaxing bath with beautiful oils, or having a massage when you notice your body feels tight. You might meet regularly with your closest friends. You might choose to dance each month under the light of the full moon. Whatever you decide, become conscious of inviting the sacred feminine into your life.

After going through perimenopause and menopause and hitting the crone years, I've been feeling a bit detached from my sensuality. Dancing the sacral chakra made me feel sexual, sensual and totally nourished.

Andrea

After dancing the sacral chakra, my inner feminine set to work, cooking nourishing food and making my home feel more nest-like. Dreams of planting flowers for Mother's Day came to me.

Suzanne

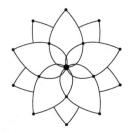

CHAPTER TWENTY-THREE

the FEMININE SHADOW

As we bring our sacral chakra into balance, we become increasingly conscious of the aspects of the feminine that we have denied within ourselves. These may be the parts of us that we felt we needed to hide to be accepted by our family or culture, like our wildness or our sensuality. Or we may have had experiences, impulses, desires or feelings that we found so embarrassing, humiliating or even terrifying that the only way we could deal with them was to bury them deep in our unconscious. These hidden parts of ourselves are what Carl Jung named our 'shadow.'

Because our shadow is hidden from our conscious life, we assume it doesn't exist. And yet the truth is that our unconscious shadow is just like the dark reflection that walks alongside us on a sunlit street—it's always dancing alongside us, whether we can see it or not. The longer we deny these hidden parts of ourselves, the more they fester and cause havoc in our lives.

Our shadow shows up as the sudden eruptions in our lives, much like a force trying to break through. It's the emotions that explode seemingly out of nowhere, which we may not even understand. It's our dark moods, our psychosomatic illnesses and, at the most extreme, those unconsciously inspired 'accidents' in our lives. If we refuse to acknowledge this dark side of our nature, it will act out unconsciously and often with great force. Balancing the sacral chakra involves bringing our feminine shadow into the light and integrating her into our lives.

At first I found the idea of accepting my shadow a frightening concept. Why would I want to dredge up the darkness within myself? Wouldn't that turn me into the person I despised and feared the most? The paradox is that the more we remain unconscious or in denial of these hidden parts of ourselves, the more force they have in our lives.

For example, we may have consciously spent our life trying to be the good girl or the nice girl, always trying to please everyone else so that we would be loved. To achieve this, we unconsciously buried our wildness, our opinions, our deep feelings. Embracing the shadow in this instance is not about suddenly becoming the bad girl. It's not about becoming a crazy, feral woman, who shouts and screams about how she feels or indulges in every dark desire. Embracing the shadow means accepting that we have our own nature, our own opinions, and our own deep feelings. Doing so shows us that we are not the good girl or the bad girl; we simply possess thoughts, feelings and drives that come and go.

However if left to fester, the shadow does behave like the bad girl—the feral, volatile woman who has been set loose in our lives. She might show up as an addiction, where we can secretly misbehave. She might explode in anger or judgement at the most inappropriate times. She might create the fantasies we are having about walking out on our partner.

Accepting our shadow allows us to take full responsibility for ourselves. Once we truly acknowledge our shadow, it will stop having control over us.

By definition our shadow is unseen, so it can be very challenging to identify those hidden parts of ourselves, especially since we have worked so hard to keep them locked away. One of the main ways we stay cut off from these parts of ourselves is by projecting them onto others—our neighbours, different cultures, those who we feel are very different to us. We can begin to recognise our shadow by noticing when we have extreme reactions to other people's behaviours or characteristics. When we disown a part of ourselves, we see it magnified in others. For example, if we have rejected our own sexuality, then overt sexuality in others will make us feel extremely uncomfortable, fearful or even repulsed. If we have buried our emotions, we will despise people who burst into tears at every drama in their lives. We can look for the hidden parts of ourselves in our extreme reactions to others.

Anne had always had an extreme reaction to overtly sexual women. Any woman who was dressed provocatively or was highly flirtatious caused an intense feeling of discomfort in her. She herself dressed very modestly and felt disconnected from her own sexuality and sensuality. When she was younger, Anne had experienced several incidents when she was violated by men. These experiences had caused her to unconsciously shut down her sexual energy, to avoid attracting unwanted attention or even violence.

When Anne danced the sacral chakra, she felt as though she was performing. At times it felt like she was outside of herself looking in. In one of her dances, she felt like parts of her were made of ice. These frozen parts made her feel like she was wearing body armour, which felt tight and restrictive. Suddenly in the dance, the frozen ice shattered. She stopped dancing and stood still, feeling the rawness of her feminine, sexual energy. She felt so different. Her movements then became wild and free, and rivers of tears began to flow. She felt like she was meeting a part of herself that she had long forgotten. The more Anne danced the sacral chakra, the more she noticed the changes in her life. She felt safer in her own sexuality. Her creativity began to flow. She felt more relaxed and able to go with the flow, without the need to try and control everything around her. As she accepted parts of herself that had previously been denied, her extreme reaction to the sexuality of other women began to fade.

Buried in our shadow are also aspects of ourselves that we perceive as positive traits in others. We may have grown up playing the pretty girl who wasn't smart, as a way of fitting in. Over the years, our inner smart girl was banished into shadow, only to be reflected back to us in the extreme admiration or envy we felt towards the clever women we encountered in our lives. The more we embrace our shadow, the more we discover the full richness of what lives within us.

Meditation: *Meet Your Inner Feminine*

You may want to try this guided meditation, as a way of connecting with different aspects of the feminine within you. You may encounter parts of you that you know and you may meet the faces of your shadow.

I have done this meditation many times over the years and have met many faces of the feminine within me. I have met both the wounded parts and the tender, graceful parts of me. I invite you to try it for yourself. Like me, you may return to this meditation many times and meet many feminine aspects of yourself.

You can do this meditation by reading the following steps, pausing after each one to imagine what has been described, or by listening to it with my voice-over guidance on the Sacral Meditation: Meet Your Inner Feminine track: [refer to page vi]

1. Prepare your sacred space and yourself. Take three slow, deep breaths.

2. Close your eyes and picture yourself sitting in your house relaxing. You hear a knock at the front door. When you open the door, everything outside looks different. It is night-time and the sky is lit up with the glow of a full moon.

3. A few steps away is a lake, with a small rowboat waiting for you. There is a safe but magical feeling in the air. You pull the boat easily into the lake, hop in, and begin to row.

4. As you move across the water in the moonlight, you see land in the distance. As you get closer to the land, you see a person waiting to greet you. You can only see the person's outline at first. As you get closer, you see that it is a woman and she is waiting for you. You reach the shore, and the woman helps you out of the boat. You now stand looking at each other and you are drawn to her eyes.

5. Notice how you are feeling as you stand with this woman. Does she have a message for you? Spend some time just being with her. The woman has a gift for you. Accept the gift and thank her.

6. It is now time to leave. You get in the boat and row back to your front door. You enter and are now back relaxing in your home. Take three deep breaths and slowly open your eyes.

Don't worry if you don't feel or see much. By simply doing this ritual, you are invoking the sacred feminine within. She will answer. She might visit you in your dreams. You may see her face in the women you encounter in your day-to-day life. Look out for her. Once invoked, she will respond to your call.

I encourage you to also try this meditation just before dancing the sacral chakra, so that you can bring the image of this feminine energy into your dance. Feel her energy merging with yours. Let her move your body. Dance her dance. She is you. I have found that each aspect of the feminine comes with a gift or a message, and it comes to you when you need it most. Feel the message in your movements and your feelings, and let that message step out with you into your life.

I have been carrying anger and sadness about my relationship not working out with my daughter's father. As I danced the sacral chakra, my buried feelings began to surface. I realise that I feel like an idiot for choosing a man who refused to be my partner when I got pregnant. I can feel how much I want my life to look good to other people. I recognise that I'm not fully owning everything about my life. As I danced, I saw myself standing in front of a big urn. I grabbed gold light from inside the urn and sprinkled it on my head. Then a dark shadow appeared. At first I felt scared. Then I heard a voice say: 'It's time to embrace your darkness.' As I danced with the shadow, it morphed into me.

Sheridan

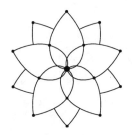

CHAPTER TWENTY-FOUR

MOVING YOUR EMOTIONS

*After dancing the sacral chakra, I have a lot of
suppressed feelings and emotions surfacing. All I can
do is give myself permission to feel, witness and honour
them as they wash over me. I found myself going
with the flow much more after dancing this chakra.*

Rhiannon

Balancing the sacral chakra helps us to feel and express our emotions in a healthy way. Our emotions are meant to flow freely. Joy, anger, fear and sadness are all natural feelings to have in response to certain situations. When we express our emotions, movement comes naturally. When we are angry, our movements can be sharp and strong. When we are nervous or anxious, our body shakes. Sadness can move through us with slow, heavy sighs.

Unfortunately, from an early age many of us were taught to stop the natural flow of our emotions. As soon as we cried, a pacifier or food was given to us to stop us crying. Our temper tantrums were thwarted mid-flow. We may have been told to sit still, when we were bursting with excitement. We learnt that expressing how we feel is not acceptable, so we began the pattern of blocking our feelings. Psychologically, we buried them in our shadow. Physically, we buried them in our bodies.

For example, perhaps we have buried our anger because we received the message that to get angry is somehow wrong. Our blocked anger tenses our physical body, as we hold it tightly in our muscles. Our dreams become violent and aggressive, as our internalised anger rages as we sleep. We live in constant fear of encountering anger out there in the world, because we are so fearful of the anger within. We sometimes find ourselves totally losing it and lashing out without any control. We feel as though we don't know what came over us.

What came over us was our anger. The deeper and longer we bury it, the more destructive it becomes as it takes on a life of its own. We find ourselves feeling exhausted by the pressure of holding this force down. If we wish to find freedom in our lives, we need to gently release our buried emotions. Movement is a natural way to do this.

When Katie danced the sacral chakra, she felt heavy and burdened. As she kept dancing, she had the image of diving into water. All the heaviness effortlessly began to melt and disperse. As she let go, she found herself crying, as she remembered an old wound she thought she had let go of many years earlier. She had the insight that her feminine sense of power, choice and vibrancy had been closed off, when she experienced date rape in her teens. She realised that she had never cried about it or really grieved over the loss of her innocence. As she danced, she felt the sadness and grief move through her. She could feel her sacral energy freeing up. She felt her choice, gentle power and sweet vibrancy return.

As you dance the sacral chakra, have the intention of allowing your body to soften and flow like water. As you physically flow, so will the feelings buried in your body, so they can be released gently. Sadness, anger, grief or excitement may wash through you as you move. Remember to let it go. Let it release. Let it move through you. You may have a memory or a vision as you dance, giving you insight into the source of the blocked emotion. Or you may just feel the emotion as it passes through you. As your feelings move, you will feel freer. You will feel the aliveness in your body and, dance by dance, you will bring forth your shadow feelings into the light.

Time to try: *The Wave*

We can help release our stuck emotions by opening our bodies and intentionally letting go, in all the places where we feel ourselves holding onto something. This simple movement called The Wave can help us soften and let go:

1. Stand with your feet hip distance apart. Softly close your eyes and take three deep breaths.

2. Lift your arms up high into the sky, and have the intention of opening up and expanding the front of your body. Next bend your knees and use your arms and body to sweep down towards the earth, like a wave sweeping down to the shore. Breathe in and lift back up like a swelling wave. Then breathe out, sweeping down and releasing as you exhale.

3. Have the intention of releasing and moving any emotions and feelings you are holding in your body.

4. Spend some time repeating the wave and finding your own rhythm. You may release even further by making sounds as you move.

5. When you have finished, you may want to journal or take some time to reflect on how you feel. Also, pay attention to what happens in your life after you have released some blocked feelings.

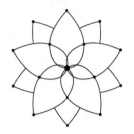

CHAPTER TWENTY-FIVE

DANCING WITH EROS

One of the beautiful gifts of dancing the sacral chakra is when we find ourselves dancing with eros. This happens when we experience the natural joy of being in our physical body, accessing our erotic nature and feelings of pleasure, and being in touch with our senses.

Eros is the life-force energy of attraction. When eros is dancing in our lives, it's not just about sex; it's the pleasurable energy that ripples through many aspects of our lives. Eros is present when we take delight in the smell of a rose, when we are moved by haunting music, when we tenderly touch our partner's skin. Our erotic nature is the aliveness of our senses, the wonderment of our bodies, the excitement of attraction. To truly embrace eros, we need to surrender to this force.

Kali had attended a Tantra workshop with two of her friends, after which they decided to go skinny-dipping in the ocean in full moonlight. Her friends were so free, happy and open, but Kali felt resistant. She found herself holding back, unable to let go as she wanted to. Months later, as she danced the sacral chakra, she found herself back in the moonlight, dancing in the waves with her friends. As she danced, she was finally able to surrender to the pure bliss and pleasure they were experiencing. She found it beautiful.

Our authentic sexuality is sensual, pure, divine and sacred. And yet, most of us are exposed to so many confusing messages about our sexuality as we grow up, especially women. Many of us have had relationships or experiences that have wounded us in some way. On top of that, we have been bombarded with distorted images and ideas about female sexuality.

Because of these messages, experiences and distortions, we tend to have a whole party going on in our unconscious, when it comes to the parts of our sexuality that we have sent into shadow. Deep within us, we have a yearning, a longing to return to our pure and divine sensual nature. We are meant to have a pleasurable connection with our own bodies. We are naturally sensual and erotic beings. This sacred energy resides within us. Balancing this chakra is about removing the layers of conditioning, unbinding the negative experiences we have had, and releasing the traumas from our stiff bodies. If we keep peeling back the layers, we will return to an inner sanctum, and this is where we will rediscover our pure and sensual nature.

As Rebecca danced the sacral chakra, she felt as though she was deep under water. Then she began to sweat, as she felt energy pouring from her sacral chakra. It was like a lightning bolt had struck her sacral chakra and was unblocking her sensual, feminine energy. Rebecca had suffered sexual abuse as a child and her experience of the dance was as if she were discovering her hidden self, her shadow, and bringing it into the light for healing. In the days following the dance, she had vivid dreams and found herself breaking into tears. It wasn't always easy, but dancing the sacral chakra began a healing process that has allowed sensual and sexual love back into her life.

When Beth danced the sacral chakra, she encountered a dark mermaid or siren from the depths of the water. This creature wasn't pretty, gentle or sweet. She was angry. She felt like the shadow of Beth's sexual self, like the embodiment of every time Beth had given away her sexual power, denied it, exploited it or failed to recognise it as sacred. Beth let this feeling move through her body. She danced and released her anger and then felt herself reclaiming her sacred sexuality.

Time to try: *Your Inner Temple*

I think of the sacral chakra as an inner temple: our own sacred inner sanctum. To reclaim our sacred sexuality, we need to heal this inner space and remember our pure and divine sensual nature.

You may want to try this exercise as a way of healing your sacred womb, the container for all of your desires, feelings and pleasure:

1. Close your eyes and imagine yourself travelling into your inner temple. What does it feel like? Is there anything you would like to bring in or take out? Does it need more colour? More beauty? Use your imagination to create the most beautiful, sensual and nourishing temple for you. You may choose to fill it with sensual music, waterfalls, or the fragrance of exotic flowers.
2. Spend some time feeling the energy in this space. Set an intention of honouring and respecting this sacred part of you.
3. To complete this exercise, I encourage you to find a creative way to reflect your inner temple in your outer world. You may choose to create a space in your home that has the same feeling. Anything that links the inner and the outer worlds is

key. It doesn't have to be a big project; it can be as simple as picking a flower or wearing a coloured scarf that feels connected to the energy in some way.

I'm apprehensive about sharing my first sacral dance, almost embarrassed. I was experiencing profound feelings of desire, sensuality and sexuality. I was this wavy, seductive temptress, almost snaky and warm. It felt like all of my body was just breathing these feelings and with the sense of water running through me. I saw images of a wild gypsy woman, seductive and tempting, but also the feeling of a lighter energy of love and sensuality. Frankly, I'm a bit surprised and timid about this really strong energy that emerged.

Cecilie

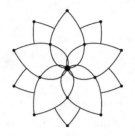

CHAPTER TWENTY-SIX

DANCING the
SACRAL CHAKRA

*The dance of the sacral chakra made me realise
that I long for deeper intimacy in my marriage.
I had a long conversation with my husband
after this experience and we have improved
the sweetness of our sexual relationship.*

Zabeth

It is now time to move your sacral chakra. Create your sacred
space and prepare yourself for your dance. Once you are ready,
begin by taking three slow, deep breaths and bringing your awareness to your lower belly and hips.

You may want to begin your movement by placing your hands
on your hips and softly bending your knees, while moving your
hips in a clockwise direction. Inhale as your hips move back and
exhale as your hips move forward. Sink deeper and deeper into

the rotations. Feel your movements becoming more fluid and loose. As you exhale, imagine releasing and letting go. Let any natural sounds or images come. You may wish to imagine you are inhaling a bright orange light. Then, as you exhale, see the release as a grey mist leaving your body. When you feel ready, change to a counter-clockwise direction. Finally, move in both directions, creating a figure eight with your hips.

When you are ready, play the music Move Your Sacral Chakra [refer to page vi] and feel the vibration of the crystal bowl pulsing at your sacral chakra. Imagine you are by the ocean under a luminous full moon. Your dance may be slow and sensual, or flirtatious and erotic, with fluid movements of the hips and lower belly. You may find yourself transforming into a wild gypsy, a belly dancer or an ancient goddess, as you surrender to the serpentine movements of the feminine.

Once you have finished your dance, take three slow, deep breaths, then sit down to create your mandala art.

Chanting the sacral chakra

The mantra sound for the sacral chakra is VAM, which is pronounced as VUM. You might like to try chanting this sound to help activate your sacral chakra.

Sit peacefully and bring your awareness to your breathing. Inhale fully through your nose. As you exhale, vocalise the mantra VAM while focusing your awareness just above your pubic bone. I recommend chanting for around five minutes, or however long feels right for you.

Take notice of any feelings, memories, images or sensations that come up for you as you chant. Spend a few minutes coming back to your natural breathing to finish.

For more information on chanting the chakras, please see Chapter 44: Sacred Singing and Chanting.

Sacral chakra affirmation: *I am sensual and passionate. My sexual energy is sacred.*

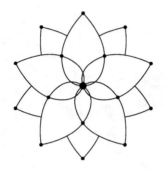

PART 5

MOVING YOUR SOLAR PLEXUS CHAKRA

*When I danced the solar plexus chakra, the
energy I experienced was immense.
I received the lesson to trust and own my power.
Not to make myself small. Roar like a lion.
Transform like the phoenix. Fight
for the good in this world.*

Maria

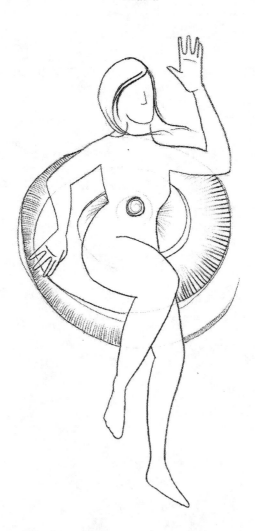

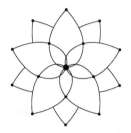

CHAPTER TWENTY-SEVEN

the SACRED MASCULINE

The solar plexus chakra is where we meet our sacred masculine. This vital energy is our inner strength, courage, self-esteem and personal power. For both women and men, allowing the sacred masculine to dance in our lives can be transformative. We learn to be driven without burning ourselves out. We learn to have authority without being controlling. We learn to stand up for ourselves without ever having to be aggressive.

When the sacred masculine begins his emergence into our lives, we feel it. We feel it in our bodies, and we experience his impact in our lives. We want to get physically fit so that we are strong, not skinny. We get clarity about the direction we want to take in our lives, and have the strength and energy to follow it through. We trust our own sense of direction, even if that means going the opposite way to everyone else. We no longer feel compelled to conform.

It's not that we are being rebellious; we are simply being authentic and following our own unique path. Sure, we may still feel fearful; but with an awakened masculine we now have an internal warrior walking through life with us. With him lighting the way, we can courageously take the risks that are sometimes needed to move ahead in our lives.

Our inner masculine connects us to our personal power. Over the years, I have led hundreds of people, predominantly women, in dancing the solar plexus chakra. I can't tell you how many of them I have seen end up in tears or in a heap on the floor, as they realise they have given away their power.

Power is such a misunderstood energy for so many of us. We travel through life having all sorts of experiences—in the schoolyard, in our relationships, workplaces, and so on. In so many of these daily interactions, we find ourselves participating in a dance of power. Who's gaining power by being dominant or, in its worst manifestation, aggressive and bullying? Who's losing power by being submissive and perhaps controlled? This dance is being played out in our lives, to a greater or lesser degree, all the time.

When I speak of reclaiming our personal power, I don't mean that we do so by gaining power over another. In fact, the power I am talking about has nothing to do with anyone else. This is the power within each of us, our personal empowerment, our internal warrior. In reclaiming our own power, we need to unravel the old patterns of how we interact with others. We also need to travel into our inner world, in order to meet and embody our masculine warrior energy.

A warrior is strong but not aggressive. Just picture a true warrior for a moment. He has incredible power but he does not go out attacking other people (physically, emotionally or verbally) to make himself feel stronger. He doesn't need to, because his strength is internal. However, if someone tries to attack him he will defend himself, but fairly and with integrity. He has a quiet self-esteem and inner confidence.

When we learn to embody our warrior energy, we radiate an inner, authentic power. We speak directly and truthfully, but with kindness. We stand up for what we believe in without putting anyone else down. We courageously follow our path, but are gentle with others as we travel. We fearlessly walk away from disrespect, but wish no harm in return. We have self-worth and we value others. We have firm boundaries, but we are open to spontaneity. This is the powerful energy of the sacred masculine.

Sherri felt like she had given her power away for most of her life, because she didn't trust herself to make the best choices. She had always hidden behind others, mostly her husband, leaving him to make the decisions for her and their family.

As Sherri danced the solar plexus chakra, she felt a tightness in her stomach. As she danced some more, she realised that this tightness was there almost all the time. She started shaking, flailing, twisting, jumping and stomping. She saw herself dancing with warriors like the Maori of New Zealand and found herself making low, strong grunting sounds that emanated from her solar plexus. She moved into elbow strikes and punches and then felt drawn to open her hands, palms up towards the sky. She saw flames rising from them and let them release. By the end of the dance her mouth was hanging open, her jaw was relaxed, and she felt like she had broken through the tightness. She finished the dance feeling determined to work through her fear and stop hiding, so that she could live her life more fully.

When Suzanne danced the solar plexus chakra, she was in the midst of tough negotiations with her business partners. She hadn't established any boundaries in these negotiations and, as a result, her partners were setting the agenda. She felt as though her understanding nature was being bullied and taken advantage of. As she danced, she was reminded to step into her power, to realise her worth and not allow others to treat her in a condescending or patronising manner. She then danced with such strength, seeing herself with bow and arrow, strong and independent, riding on a powerful horse. She felt as though her inner warrior princess was back on her game. She took this energy into her meetings with her business partners, and it helped a lot with her negotiations.

Time to try: *Reclaiming Your Personal Power*

We can begin reclaiming our personal power by consciously looking at our lives and being honest about our own power struggles. Use the following questions to help you gain some insight:

1. Sit down with a piece of paper and pen and write down answers to the following questions: Are there any noticeable power struggles going on in my life at the moment? What could I do to change them?
2. Spend some time tuning into the most important relationships in your life—your partner, children, parents, friends, work colleagues, etc. Then ask yourself: How does each relationship make me feel? Am I in my authentic power in each of these relationships?

Once you've found areas of your life that are out of balance in this way, I suggest working on one dynamic at a time, beginning with small steps towards making changes. For example, if your work colleague is often rude or dismissive with you and you normally say nothing in return, perhaps it's time to be more truthful about how you would like to be treated. Step into your warrior energy and you will be able to speak your truth, but with kindness. Or maybe you are too controlling and bossy with your children. It may be time to find encouraging ways to teach them how to take more responsibility.

These shifts take practice, patience and diligence. They work best when we go through our power dynamics one by one, shining a spotlight on what is actually happening in our lives. Most of the time we are so stuck in old habits that we're not even conscious of how the dynamics are playing out in our relationships. If we want to find freedom in our lives, we need to clarify how we operate, then consciously make necessary changes.

This exercise can be challenging. When there is a particular power dynamic between two people (or a group of people) and one person starts changing the dance, it can cause a higher level of pain for a while. The other person may unconsciously crave the safety of the old dynamic and begin to exaggerate their behaviour, as a way of coaxing you back into the old pattern. Remain consistent, persistent and centred in your warrior power.

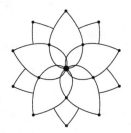

CHAPTER TWENTY-EIGHT

LIVING a WARRIOR LIFE

Many years ago, I came across a quote by Marian Woodman, Jungian analyst and author, whose writing resonates deeply with me. She said: *When you let go of the shell that covers your true nature, you discover the radiance of your authentic self.*

These words have resonated with me when working on my own solar plexus chakra, and I have been reminded of them often when working with others to balance theirs. We all have our true radiance, strength and warrior energy within us. It never really goes away. When we feel as though we have lost it, that's because it has been covered up in some way. Our shell may be our own critical voice or criticism from another that we have taken on. It may be our own harsh judgements or beliefs about ourselves. It may result from an early trauma we've experienced. When we are able to let this shell go, to release it, we can own our true power again.

Natasha runs her own small business and came to Chakradance because she was feeling burnt out. She had grown up believing that her power was something she needed to push for, work hard for, even fight for. She would charge out into the world and become very controlling, forcing her way through situations to get what she wanted. Because this took up so much energy, she would end up exhausted and defeated, which often caused her to give up. This was the cycle that she became stuck in, moving from one extreme to the other.

Dancing the solar plexus chakra revealed to Natasha that she wasn't owning or even connecting with her true inner power. She was trying to find it outside herself. She could also see how critical of herself she was. She hadn't completed high school and her deep feelings of inadequacy were affecting how she lived her life. The more she danced the solar plexus chakra, the more she realised her own self-worth. She was able to see all she has achieved and her self-esteem grew. She no longer approaches her work, or her life, in the same way. She has changed the old pattern. Natasha now radiates an inner confidence. As a result, her business and her life are flourishing.

When we connect with our authentic power, we don't need to push, force or manipulate. We don't need to feel defeated or exhausted. The warrior energy within us is a gentle yet potent power. It's like a strong flame that never dies. From this place, we can move mountains when we need to, and we can do it almost effortlessly. The warrior energy is always available to us. The key is to remove the blocks that are impeding our connection with our inner power.

Responding to challenges as a warrior

Throughout our lives, we will be confronted with challenging situations. All the dancing in the world is not going to stop that from happening. We have no real control over what comes at us, but we do have control over how we respond. We can either be defeated and taken down by our challenges, or we can stand true in our own power and respond from a place of authentic strength. Feelings like self-doubt may still surface; but with a strong solar plexus energy. we can acknowledge them and choose to respond from the energy of the warrior.

A few years ago, I experienced a chain of events that brought many aspects of my life crashing down around me. My initial reaction was to crumble and feel weak and hopeless. It was a scary time, and I really felt like I had lost my power to events totally out of my control. In hindsight, I can see that this time brought me enormous growth. I began dancing the solar plexus chakra every morning. Each day I felt a little more connected to my inner strength, my own energy, my internal power. Even though chaos was going on around me, I started to deal with it from a place of strength that I had never truly known. I calmly took responsibility for making some huge decisions and took action on things that needed doing. Every now and then I would get a wave of 'I can't do this—I'm not strong enough' or 'poor me!' But then I would return to that inner strength and keep moving forwards.

This chapter of my life really helped me find my authentic power. It felt like a painful way to discover it, but I am grateful for what I've learnt.

I still have times when I feel defeated or powerless or lose my confidence or self-esteem, but it's never for long. I now find myself reconnecting back to my inner warrior quite quickly. I trust that my inner strength is always there. For me, this is one of the biggest gifts to come from dancing the solar plexus chakra.

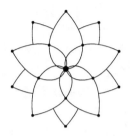

CHAPTER TWENTY-NINE

the MASCULINE SHADOW

Sadly, many of us have a fear of the masculine. When this energy is out of balance, it can lead to aggression and violence, so it's no wonder that we can become fearful of it.

When Pamela danced the solar plexus chakra for the first time, she discovered her deep fear of masculine energy. It felt to her like this energy would unleash war, pain and hurt on humanity. She then had the insight that this had also been her experience of males in her world. She knew it was time to release these experiences and invoke the sacred masculine energy within.

The aggression and violence in our world is a reflection of the darkest shadow of the masculine. It's only natural that we sometimes shut down our masculine energy in fear, or even respond to aggression with excessive force. This is why a return to an awakened sacred masculine is so necessary. As we connect with our true warrior energy, it not only helps us find freedom—it also creates freedom in the world around us.

Throughout my life I have done various forms of martial arts, including karate and chi gung (aka qi gong). These practices have taught me a lot about the true nature of the masculine. He is our deep integrity, our willpower and our strength. He is our dedication, decisiveness and unwavering commitment to our journey. Without a doubt, the sacred masculine is a strong and powerful force. It's a vital energy that we all need to embody, if we are to get out there and do the amazing work we are here to do. We need the masculine, so that we can courageously follow our true path.

When Teneisha first danced the solar plexus chakra, she found it difficult to express her inner masculine, compared to the feminine flow of her sacral chakra. Her movements felt uncertain, choppy and awkward. She wanted to remain beautiful, composed and womanly, rather than get crazy and aggressive. As she continued to dance, she saw a brilliant topaz jewel implanted in her upper belly, shining like a lighthouse. She had visions of herself as a crusader knight, a shaman in the Amazon, and a Native American warrior dancing around a fire after a hunt. She realised then that she needed to strengthen her solar plexus, to take up space and hold her ground. The dance showed her that she can be a woman and still channel masculine power.

Just as with the feminine, part of reclaiming the sacred masculine is to restore the parts of him that we have disowned. We may have been told we were too bossy when we were growing up, so now have difficulty asserting authority. Perhaps we didn't like the negative attention of being too smart, so we stopped trying hard to achieve. We may have buried aspects of our inner 'he' so deeply that we no longer even recognise them. Instead, we might project him onto the people in our lives, and he visits us as male figures in our dreams.

Take notice of what causes extreme reactions in you, both positive and negative. We have a tendency to project our disowned strengths and the parts of us that we can't bear to identify with. Consciously notice when your extreme idealisations or overwhelming reactions come up. What is the message that is being reflected back to you? Remember, the more we banish aspects of ourselves into shadow, the less control we have over how they impact on our lives.

Meditation: *Meet Your Inner Masculine*

Try the following guided meditation, as a way of connecting with the different aspects of the masculine within you. You may encounter parts that you know and you may meet faces of your shadow. You may, like me, return to this meditation many times and meet the many masculine aspects of you.

You can do this meditation by reading the following steps, pausing after each one to imagine what has been described, or by listening to it with my voice-over guidance on the Solar Plexus Meditation: Meet Your Inner Masculine track: [refer to page vi]

1. Prepare your sacred space and yourself. Take three slow, deep breaths.
2. Softly close your eyes and picture yourself sitting in your house relaxing. You hear a knock at the front door. When you open the door, everything outside looks different. As you step outside, you find yourself on a sand dune in the middle of the desert, just before dawn. It is still quite dark, but there is a campfire burning to keep you warm.
3. As you look to the horizon, you see that the sun beginning to rise. You raise your arms in greeting, as this powerful force emerges from the darkness of the night.
4. And now, as the sun rises higher and lights the sky, you see in the distance a person slowly walking towards you. As this

person crosses the sand dunes and moves closer to you, you see that it is a man.

5. As he reaches you, he stops and sits with you next to your campfire. You now sit looking directly into each other's eyes. This man feels familiar to you somehow.

6. Notice how you feel with this man. Does he have a message for you? Spend some time just being with him. The man has a gift for you. You accept the gift and thank him.

7. It is now time for you to return to your home. You turn and walk away from the fire and find yourself standing back at your front door. You enter and are now back relaxing in your home.

8. Take three deep breaths, then slowly open your eyes.

Just as with the *Meet Your Inner Feminine* meditation, don't worry if you don't feel or see much. By simply doing this ritual, you are invoking the sacred masculine within. He will respond. He might visit you in your dreams or come to you as a message through an encounter in your life.

I encourage you to also try this meditation just before dancing the solar plexus chakra, so that you can bring the image of this masculine energy into your dance. Dance his energy, as he is an aspect of you.

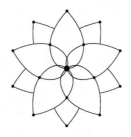

CHAPTER THIRTY

CHARGING UP YOUR LIFE

Our masculine energy needs to be embodied, because he literally energises us. He gets us out of bed and moving into the day. He gives us our direction and purpose.

For the last couple of years, Claire had been feeling drained and burnt out. Her doctor recommended that she go on sick leave, to try to pull herself together. Even though she practised lots of different therapies, she could not get out of this burnt-out state. Nothing she did seemed to give her more than a temporary reprieve.

When Claire found Chakradance, she felt a big energetic block as she danced the solar plexus chakra. She continued to dance, and gradually felt the block begin to shift. She began to feel like herself again. Since then, she has been finishing projects and decluttering her house and office. One night over the dinner table, her husband looked at her and said, 'I can feel the energy and power radiating from you. What's going on? Is Chakradance helping you?' Claire smiled and confirmed that yes, it was.

The masculine helps us break through our inertia. Quite often, people arrive at my classes saying how tired and exhausted they are from the stresses of the day. They arrive feeling like they are incapable of dancing to the wild, fiery, dynamic music of the solar plexus. Almost always, once they begin the dance, the energy of the solar plexus charges them up. It's like they have been refuelled. They leave feeling energised and full of life. This charge, this energy current, lives within us all. Dancing the solar plexus is like going to the service station for a refill.

Once we have charged ourselves up, we can channel our energy wherever it needs to go in our lives. We can finally complete that project, make that challenging decision, or take the next right action. Dancing the masculine motivates us and gives us the confidence to step out into the world and do what we need to do.

When Rebecca finished dancing the solar plexus chakra, she felt very emotional. She felt like her inner fire had only been smouldering before, and through the dance it had been brought to life. She was surprised by how emotional this made her feel, yet she also felt liberated to know that she had been the one holding herself back. She made a commitment to keep dancing, to keep those flames burning, to believe in herself, and to trust that what she wants to achieve is possible.

Time to try: *Warrior Charge*

If you find yourself feeling sluggish and tired, you might want to try this simple but very powerful exercise to recharge yourself:

1. Stand up and come into a warrior position—feet wide apart and knees bent, so that you are squatting. Cross your arms and lift your elbows out straight in front of you. Sink your

knees a little deeper. Spend a few moments in this warrior position and notice how you feel. What's your energy like?

2. Now, drop your arms but keep your knees bent. Use your breath and your hands to push out any stagnant energy.

3. Exaggerate your breath and, on each exhalation, push your hands out with the intention of releasing any tired or sluggish energy. Now use sound to release further. As you push your hands out, make the sound HA, or any sound that helps you release stuck energy. Keep releasing for as long as feels right for you.

4. Come back into the original warrior position—knees bent, arms crossed and elbows straight in front of you. Once again, notice how you feel. What's your energy like now?

5. Take three deep breaths, and step out into your day feeling energised and clear.

This simple exercise can make such a difference to our energy levels in just a few short minutes. Keep it in your chakra toolkit and try it out at different times. If you do it first thing in the morning, it can make a difference to how your whole day unfolds. If you sit at a desk all day and start to feel drained by the afternoon, try it out during your afternoon slump. Always remember: the masculine is our fuel.

I arrived at the solar plexus chakra feeling tired and exhausted. But when I got into this warrior dance, my body moved in such fast and forceful movements I couldn't stop it. It was as if it had its own will.

Catherine

*Avoiding ... that is how I started out with the
solar plexus dance. I put the music on but walked
around, fed the kitties, looked at Facebook. Then
it started. The music was boiling up and I started
vibrating—hands, feet, my whole body, every
part of me vibrating. I was on fire. I was the fire,
fully alive flames emanating from every pore.
Releasing, alive, glowing and so full of life force.*

Corina

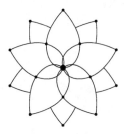

CHAPTER THIRTY-ONE

BURNING it AWAY

The dance of the solar plexus is a fiery dance. In many ways, it is a dance of transformation. This dance reminds me of a story from Greek mythology: the phoenix rising from the ashes. The phoenix is a mythical bird that lives for up to 100 years. At the end of its life, it settles into its nest and burns ferociously. Both bird and nest turn to ashes. From those ashes, a new phoenix rises. It's like a rebirth.

The dance of the solar plexus is our opportunity to burn away all that no longer serves us, to release the judgements, the outdated beliefs, the critical voices, so that we can once again feel our inner power radiate outwards. Through this dance, we can have our own rebirth.

Before dancing the solar plexus chakra, Rhiannon sat quietly and asked herself: 'What do I need to burn away in this dance? What do I no longer need? What is no longer serving me? What is holding me back from empowering myself? What is it within me that depletes my energy levels?'

She then allowed herself to be completely honest. She wrote a list of what she wanted to burn during the dance. She wanted to release her jealousy, her envy of strong and confident women, and her awkward shyness. She wanted to burn away her fear of meeting new people, her tendency not to recognise her own self-worth, and her belief that other people were better than her. She wanted to release all this silly nonsense and negative self-talk, so she could step into her true warrior self.

Rhiannon's dance was one of the most freeing experiences she'd ever had. She finally felt like the hero of her own life.

Before dancing your solar plexus chakra, I encourage you to write a list of what you need to burn away in order to connect with your inner power, just like Rhiannon did. What is holding you back? What beliefs do you have about yourself that are not serving you? What ways of thinking are depleting your energy? Get real with yourself. This is not about judgement; it's about identifying what the shell covering your authentic power is made of. You can then burn away this shell during your dance.

As Pippa danced the solar plexus chakra, she saw the image of a flame building into a massive fire. She flicked all her negativity into the fire and it grew and grew, burning it all away. She continued to dance and then she saw the image of a powerful Indian chief. She threw spears and drummed with this Indian chief, to celebrate her inner feeling of power.

As Moira danced, she began to see dark images. She felt envy and jealousy surface and then heard an inner voice say, 'Let it all go.' She heard words of judgement and criticism, followed by whispers of release. She was sweating more and more as she continued to release. Towards the end of the dance, an image of a huge, handsome man appeared and the name Thor came to her.

She felt like she had a gentle volcano centred in her being. She had found her power.

Time to try: *Breath of Fire*

The breath of fire is a powerful breathing technique. As you practise this breath, feel your inner fire building in your solar plexus and have the intention of burning away anything that no longer serves you:

1. Place your hands on your lower belly. As you breathe in through your nose, your lungs fill with air and your belly pushes out. Feel your belly pushing into your hands. As you exhale through your nose, empty your lungs and flatten your belly. At the end of your exhalation, gently pull your navel towards your spine.

2. Once again, breathe in gently through your nose, feeling your belly expand. Exhale through your nose as you press your navel towards your spine, gently using your abdominal muscles. Begin doing this quickly, almost like a dog panting, only through your nose instead of your mouth. Feel your belly bounce.

3. Do this rapid breathing about thirty times, making sure that you breathe in and out of your nose each time. If you feel comfortable with this breathing, you can repeat the cycle of thirty breaths up to four times.

4. To finish, return to your normal breathing and feel your power, energy and strength.

As I danced the solar plexus chakra, the flickering and growing flames burned me up and I welcomed their transforming energy. Shaking this off was instinctual and necessary, a feeling of toxic release.

Jessica

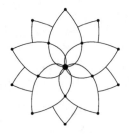

CHAPTER THIRTY-TWO

SACRED BOUNDARIES

Another gift that comes from embodying the sacred masculine is learning to have boundaries. Brené Brown, research professor and speaker, talks about how thirteen years of research confirmed that the most compassionate people are those who have good, clear boundaries. She describes boundaries quite simply as: *What's okay, and what's not okay.*

Many of us have grown up trying to please others, out of a desperate desire to be liked. We avoid conflict and confrontation, because it makes us feel uncomfortable or even fearful. As a result, we go through life letting people do things or behave in ways that are not okay with us. Each time this not-okay behaviour happens, we don't confront it. Instead, we end up silently resenting or even hating the other person. This toxic energy burns away inside us, making us feel disrespected and angry.

Throughout my life, I have struggled with setting boundaries. Many years ago, a friend asked if he and his girlfriend could stay with my husband and me for a week. I didn't really want them to stay as I was busy with work, but I didn't want to upset anyone so I agreed. When they arrived, the girlfriend settled into our home very much like it was her own. She helped herself to everything in the house, including my bathroom toiletries. Inside I didn't feel that this was okay, but as I didn't want to upset my friend or cause a scene, I didn't say anything.

One evening, we met them at a restaurant for dinner. As they walked in, I recognised the dress the girlfriend was wearing. Then I looked down and realised that I also recognised the shoes. In a very tight voice I asked her about them, and she said that she had taken them from my closet. I sat there seething all night, still saying nothing. I became very cold and removed during the rest of their stay, and I haven't seen them since. By not having boundaries, I cost myself a week of stress, ended up in a hostile situation, and may have even lost a friend as a result.

Connecting with the sacred masculine has taught me how to have sacred boundaries. I call them 'sacred' because I can now see how they are a form of self-love and respect. Respect not only for myself, but also for the person or people I am setting the boundaries with. If I had been clear about what was okay from the beginning, then my friend and his girlfriend wouldn't even have been staying with me, let alone getting into my things. Or if I had set house rules, then perhaps their stay would have been more enjoyable for everyone.

I have now become much better at saying 'no.' The 'no' comes from such a deep and authentic place within me that it almost holds its own vibration. It's not aggressive, it's powerful. I no longer come across as sweet and soft as I used to, but I'm far more authentic and therefore less critical and judgemental. I'm also happier.

Healing broken boundaries

If the boundaries that should be our natural human right are broken when we are young, before we have the power within us to insist on them, we can be left carrying that trauma throughout our lives.

When Gwen was five years old, she experienced a sexual trauma. This violation had a massive impact on her. She went into a frozen state, buried her anger, and was left feeling like a victim. She has carried those feelings throughout her life.

When Gwen danced the solar plexus chakra, she instinctively began throwing energy off herself. She felt as though she were releasing the victim energy she had been carrying. She then began stomping around the room forcefully, as her inner warrior demanded to make himself known. He made his presence known through big movements and loud exhalations of breath. She could feel her strength and power. It was like she was reclaiming some of her lost energy. She then experienced waves of anger. Sometimes it felt like that anger was directed inwards, sometimes outwards. She felt like she was releasing some of the anger that she carried towards her perpetrator, and some that she had carried towards herself for freezing up. She spontaneously started to cleanse her energy field. Then, she imagined energetic bricks and created a protective igloo of energy around herself. Her igloo felt like a safe space, a boundary that she had lacked since the trauma.

Energy boundaries

Just as we need to have physical and behavioural boundaries, we also need to have energy boundaries. Have you ever had friends who spent an entire night dumping all of their dramas onto you? They leave saying how much better they feel, and you leave feeling utterly exhausted.

When Magdalena danced the solar plexus chakra, she realised that she felt like a sponge. She was constantly taking on other people's problems, emotions and energy, then owning them as if they were her own. She felt as though this habit was literally sucking the energy out of her.

Some people, some situations, even some places can be like energy vampires—literally! Start to take notice of how your energy feels after being in certain places or with particular friends or colleagues. If you feel your energy dips or plummets, this is a sign that you need to set up your energy boundaries.

Time to try: *Setting Energy Boundaries*

What follows are two simple techniques for setting and reinforcing energy boundaries within your daily life.

– CALLING IN THE WHITE LIGHT

When I was studying to become an energy healer at the College of Psychic Studies, I learnt a powerful energy protection exercise that I have used every day of my life since. In this exercise, you imagine a circle of white light surrounding you and you say: *I'm surrounded by the white light of divine energy, through which nothing negative can penetrate.*

I visualise this white light and say these words before I leave the house, before entering a public space, and when I catch up with people. This energy boundary isn't a wall of separation; it is simply a way of protecting my energy. I no longer come away from vampire-like situations feeling drained. Sometimes I'll reinforce the intention while I'm out, and I've found it keeps growing in power the more I do it.

− SEALING YOUR AURA

This exercise takes only a few minutes and is a great thing to do as part of your morning meditation or ritual, as you get out of the shower or when you are brushing your teeth, so that it becomes a natural part of your life.

Begin by imagining your aura, the energy field around you, as an egg-shaped cocoon. Visualise a shaft of white light entering through the top of your head. Breathe the light all the way down to your heart chakra at the centre of your chest. As you breathe out, send the white light out through your heart and hands, filling your aura, the cocoon around you, with white light. Keep breathing in the light from above and breathing out into the cocoon. After a few minutes, visualise the outer edge of your aura becoming like an eggshell. Know that the shell will only allow positive energy to pass through. Mentally affirm that your aura is now sealed.

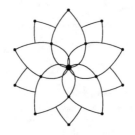

CHAPTER THIRTY-THREE

DANCING the SOLAR PLEXUS CHAKRA

This morning I danced the solar plexus chakra. It was incredible! Probably the best dance of my life. I felt so much strength, power and confidence surface during the dance. I felt like a warrior on my horse going into battle to beat self-criticism and low self-esteem. And I won!

Rhiannon

It is now time to move your solar plexus chakra. Set up your sacred space and prepare yourself for your dance. Once you are ready, begin by taking three slow, deep breaths, then bring your awareness to your solar plexus chakra (between your navel and the base of your sternum). You may feel it as an energetic space around your diaphragm. Visualise your solar plexus as a beautiful jewel, like a yellow diamond shining outwards. Imagine you are standing by an ancient campfire.

When you are ready, play the Move Your Solar Plexus Chakra music [refer to page vi] and feel the sound of the crystal bowl activating your solar plexus chakra. In this dance you may shake, vibrate, even become frenzied and wild, as you burn away all the things that are holding you back in life. You may literally move as though you are the fire. You may find yourself making strong, defined, purposeful movements, as you express the powerful energy of the sacred masculine. Your chest may lift and your shoulders may broaden as the triumphant feeling of becoming your own warrior pulses through you.

Once you have finished your dance, take three slow, deep breaths, then sit down to create your mandala art.

The angel of fire. Today's dance of the solar plexus was powerful. I really felt like I was cutting the chains of the past. My whole being was on fire. I even had a past life memory, where I saw myself chained up and powerless.

Magdalena

Dancing the solar plexus was amazing. I haven't moved like that in years. Once my feet were freed from the molten black lava that I was stuck in, I felt my power. I'm still feeling it. The fire in my belly is burning through and rising up for me to be my most powerful self.

Christine

Chanting the solar plexus chakra

The mantra sound for the solar plexus chakra is RAM, which is pronounced as RUM. You might like to try chanting this sound to help activate your solar plexus chakra.

Sit peacefully and bring your awareness to your breathing. Inhale fully through your nose. As you exhale, vocalise the mantra RAM while focusing your awareness just above your navel. I recommend chanting for around five minutes, or however long feels right for you.

Take notice of any feelings, memories, images or sensations that come to you as you chant. Spend a few minutes coming back to your natural breathing to finish.

For more information on chanting the chakras, please see Chapter 44: Sacred Singing and Chanting.

Solar plexus chakra affirmation:
I am worthy. I am powerful.
I courageously follow my own unique path.

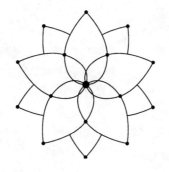

PART 6

MOVING YOUR
HEART CHAKRA

*Tonight I danced the heart chakra and felt so
connected, so light. My six-year-old daughter was
playing quietly in the room, listening to the music.
While I was dancing the heart chakra, my mother
(who passed away seventeen years ago) appeared to
me midway through, and held her arms out to me.
As she approached me I felt her say, 'It's time
to let it go, soften your heart, and let it go.'
Just as we were about to embrace, my daughter
quietly and softly came up to me, hugged me and
danced with me. I think it may have been the most
beautiful feeling my heart has felt in a very long time.*

Mary

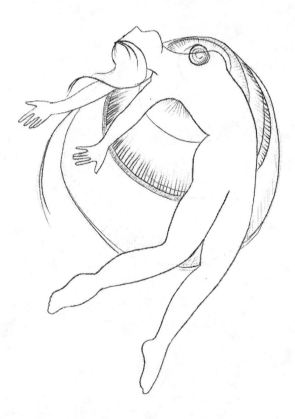

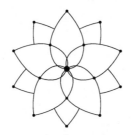

CHAPTER THIRTY-FOUR

NATURAL RHYTHMS
of the HEART

The heart chakra is one of the most beautiful chakras to engage with, as well as one of the most painful. Nothing else quite beats the feeling of being in love—with a partner, a child, the sunrise, with life itself. It feels like we are walking on air. The beauty in our lives feels exquisite. We find it easy to be joyful, kind and generous, with others and with ourselves.

However, if something happens to hurt our hearts—our partner leaves us, a parent dies, or a friend betrays us—it's as though we plummet to the depths. This is a natural human response when we experience pain in our hearts. We temporarily withdraw from the world and go through the agonising process of grieving. In many ways, the heart holds both the rose and the thorn, and we will experience both in our lives.

Our heart chakra stays balanced, if we allow ourselves to fully experience the natural rhythms of the heart. This means accepting that there will be times in our lives when we suffer. Although we don't want or need to hold onto the pain forever, it is a natural and healthy response to sometimes feel sadness in our lives. If a loved one dies, we are going to be thrown into a state of grief. If our marriage ends in divorce, we are going to feel scared and depressed. If we are diagnosed with an illness, we are going to feel a deep sadness.

Grief can be a time of extraordinary growth in our lives. When we journey through our darkest hours, we often learn a lot about ourselves and have the greatest opportunity to transform our lives. Some call this time 'the dark night of the soul.' We withdraw from the world and surrender to our pain. We are called to examine our part in the failures we have experienced. We may even have to face our own mortality. Grief is a natural process. If we allow ourselves to grieve fully, the grief will come to a natural end.

Sadly, many of us live in families or societies where we are encouraged to get over our pain too quickly. We may turn to medication to try to numb the pain. We may jump into a new relationship, to try to stop mourning the one we have just lost. We may find ourselves compulsively working or partying—whatever it takes to distance ourselves from the hurt. While we may feel that it's not natural to suffer, running away from grief doesn't make it go away. When we thwart this natural process, all we do is turn the pain inwards. We trap the sadness, the loss, the rejection, the betrayal and the shock in our bodies. We lock it all inside our broken hearts.

To truly find freedom in our lives, we need to gently begin to release the pain we have been holding onto, so that we can return to love. We can do that by dancing the heart chakra.

Caroline was eleven years old when her father died. She was living in Malaysia at the time. The moment she realised that he was dead, she thought: 'Right, if this is the way life wants to play, I'm out. I will close my heart from here on.' And she did. She never even cried. Due to his passing, she had to move with her remaining family to Holland, a country she had never lived in before. She had to part from her cats and all her friends. She felt as though she didn't only lose her father, but her whole life as she knew it. She started at a new school in Holland just a few days after her father's funeral. Her new teacher was nasty to her and she felt bullied by him. At the time, she thought that her decision to close her heart was a good one, as she really needed protection in her new situation.

As Caroline became an adult, she realised that her decision to shut down her heart had impacted negatively on her whole life. She knew she needed to release the pain of her father's death, but she didn't know how to. Also, her fear of feeling the pain was enormous.

When Caroline danced the heart chakra, she knew she had found a way. Finally, after all the years of holding them back, her tears came. Then the pain was released as sound—the deepest, purest, animal-like sound she had ever heard. She sweated and felt dizzy. Then she felt cold and was covered in goosebumps. The skin on her face tingled and her hands felt swollen. Suddenly, a white light appeared in front of her and she knew it was the soul of her father. He put his hands in hers. She could **feel** them. As well as pain, she also felt the deepest sense of happiness and joy. They danced together, holding hands. She felt so much love. She felt so comforted being with her father, after all those years of having withheld him from her heart.

Since dancing the heart chakra, Caroline's life has completely changed. She is now enjoying every minute of it. She feels so much lighter and happier. She has trained to become a Chakradance Facilitator and is going to start her own healing practice, so she can help others on their healing journey.

*As I began dancing the heart chakra, I started crying.
My tears of release intensified as I continued, and I
found myself gasping for air, almost as though I was
drowning in my pain. I realised just how much hurt I
have been carrying in my heart. I kept dancing, allowing
the feelings to move through my body. Towards the
end of the dance I felt much lighter, as though I was
flying with a bird, up high with beautiful blue ocean
waters beneath me. I began to breathe more deeply
and felt as though my heart had begun to soften.*

Cecilie

*When I danced the heart chakra, I had recently lost
my sister. As I danced, I was able to feel connected
to her. I found this dance to be a safe and powerful
way to express my grief, which at times has felt
as though it has been hemmed inside me, with its
pressure growing dangerously stronger all the time.*

Helen

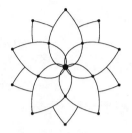

CHAPTER THIRTY-FIVE

HEALING FROM
LOSS and PAIN

The pain in our hearts is not always about the loss of a loved one or difficulty in a relationship. We can feel a deep sense of grief when our children leave home. We can feel loss when our bodies or minds can no longer perform in the way they used to. I know many people who feel a painful loss when they realise how much time they have lost on other things, when they could have been following their dreams. These losses are often held as unexpressed grief in our hearts and heaviness in our chests. As with all pain, we need to feel it and then release it, energetically and physically.

Doreen had been through several major losses over a period of seven years. First she lost her mum, then she began menopause, and then her dad passed away. She had been carrying all this pain in her heart.

When Doreen danced the heart chakra, she was drawn to dance with her arms wide open. She could feel the air moving quickly around her, as if she were taking flight. At one point, she saw herself sitting on top of a huge mountain with God and Jesus. A white dove appeared and it transformed into the Holy Spirit. She sat there overwhelmed by their presence, crying many tears. She felt like she had arrived home again after a very long journey. For the first time in a long time, she felt complete peace and joy.

Our heart chakras can become heavy when we suffer from too many burdens in our lives. You may find yourself caring for an elderly parent, as well as your own children. You may be a single mother working three jobs to support your family. When we carry a lot of burden, we often put a wall around our hearts. It's not that we are uncaring. In fact, everything we are doing is about caring for other people. The wall goes up to try to stop the pain we are feeling inside. We may be grieving for the loss of freedom and beauty in our lives, just like we would for the loss of a loved one.

A few years ago, I was invited to run a Chakradance workshop for a group of mothers who all had disabled children needing full-time physical and emotional care. I intuitively decided to run the heart chakra dance. When I arrived, I could feel the collective wall from the group. Every one of these brave women had their arms crossed, to physically and energetically protect themselves. They had spent so much of their lives holding it together that there was a real fear of what would happen if they opened up.

In the beginning, these women found it really challenging to move their bodies, because they were holding on so tightly. As the dance continued, most of them began crying softly, as they gradually let go of the pain they had been holding onto for years. They shared with me afterwards how much lighter and more connected they felt to themselves. One of the organisers of the workshop commented that they all looked like they had just been on a week's holiday.

Even when we have huge responsibilities, it's crucial that we feed and nurture our hearts for the sake of our own health. I'm reminded here of the guidance we are given when we catch a plane. We are advised in an emergency to put our own oxygen mask on first, before we help those dependent on us. We need to be fully breathing ourselves, before we can be of genuine help to others.

Healing from loss, pain or burden is not something that we have to do completely on our own. There is help available, if only we ask.

About ten years ago, I had an extraordinarily powerful experience while I was dancing the heart chakra. As I danced, the most intense, blinding light appeared, and with the light came a powerful presence I had never experienced before. I then felt two huge wings of light wrap around me, and I heard the name Uriel. I had never heard the name before; it was only later when I researched it that I realised it's the name of an angel. I was in a kind of shock while this was happening, but there was also something so pure, divine and real about it, so I didn't feel scared. I felt totally safe and very held.

Uriel asked me to hand over to him any pain or weight that I was carrying in my heart. He showed me how it had been there for too long, and that I didn't need to carry it anymore. This weight and heaviness wasn't serving me or the world. The whole experience felt like a spontaneous healing of my heart and a true blessing, albeit a bit of a surreal one.

Although I haven't had an experience as intense as that again, I now fully trust that there is angelic help available to us. I now often hand over any heaviness to the angels as I dance the heart chakra, and always feel healing and lightness when I do.

When Sherri danced the heart chakra, she started by feeling angry and her movements were heavy and jerky. She finally broke down and cried, letting it all out. She sat on the floor, held a pillow and rocked, asking why it was so hard for her to let the heaviness in her heart go. She asked if anyone was there to help her. Then she felt angels slowly moving their wings around her, sending her love and compassion. She asked the angels to take her burden from her. She gave it up and the angels lifted the heaviness from her chest. She finished the dance feeling so open and ready to move on.

Time to try: *Physically Releasing Hurt from Your Heart*

When we are holding pain in our hearts, we lock it into our bodies. Our breath becomes shallow, as it fights to flow through the many layers of protection. To find freedom, we need to release the hurt and grief from our bodies.

If you feel you are carrying pain in your heart, try this exercise:

1. Come into a standing position with your knees slightly bent. Gently lift your shoulders up and back.
2. Deepen your breathing, focusing on it as you inhale and exhale. As you breathe in, imagine drawing light into your heart. As you breathe out, have the intention of releasing the pain and hurt from your heart. Spend a few minutes doing this.
3. You may deepen your experience by imagining you are breathing different colours in and out. I often breathe in a sparkling white light and see the pain releasing as a murky grey.
4. You may have memories surface as you breathe, or see images in your mind's eye. Just observe what is happening. Don't try to control or judge it.
5. You may choose to ask yourself: 'What am I repressing? What am I holding down in my life?' Sometimes we don't know what we have been holding onto or what is making us feel

depressed. If that's the case, simply ask for whatever needs to be released to surface, then breathe it out.

6. When you are ready, begin rolling your shoulders backwards to expand and open your chest. Match the rhythm of your breathing to your movements. Have the intention of releasing any tightness in your heart and softening the holding. Keep breathing deeply, with the intention of releasing on your out-breath. Now circle your arms backwards, so that your heart is opening even wider and you are releasing even further.

7. When you are ready, place both hands over your heart and take three deep breaths. Feel the warmth of your hands pour into your heart.

> *Ahhh, the heart chakra. What can I say—*
> *it was beautiful, lyrical, yummy, delightful.*
> *I became an angel who spread a healing balm*
> *all over the world. It felt profound.*
>
> Toni

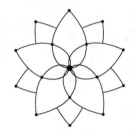

CHAPTER THIRTY-SIX

the POWER of LOVE

At the core of the heart chakra is self-love. If we are to find loving relationships with others, we need to learn to deeply love ourselves first.

Self-love is ultimately about being kind and compassionate with ourselves. Think about how you would treat a friend who is struggling or down on herself. Now think about how you treat yourself when you are feeling the same way. So often we are much kinder to others than we are to ourselves. A friend of mine started noticing that every time she is unkind to herself, she accidently trips, bumps her leg, or physically injures herself in some way. She has come to see her bruises as evidence that she is literally beating herself up.

How we love ourselves has an enormous impact on almost every aspect of our lives—from the relationships we attract, the way we cope with problems, even our physical health. If we love ourselves, we are kind to ourselves. We won't treat our bodies like machines. We won't be so hard on ourselves when we fail at something. We won't allow ourselves to be treated badly by others.

Kate has been with her partner for fifteen years. Although she loves him deeply, much of their time together has been filled with sadness. Her partner has suffered rage episodes all of his adult life, as a result of the trauma he experienced as a young child and while growing up. Kate finally found enough love for herself to say 'no more.' With the help of a highly-skilled trauma counsellor, together with the love and commitment they have for each other, Kate's partner and their relationship are healing.

When Kate danced the heart chakra, she saw herself and her partner picking up the broken pieces of her heart and putting them back together in loving kindness. She feels like her relationship is healing, and she is also healing through her journey of genuine self-love. After the dance, she gave herself a hug and could feel comfort in that. She gave her mandala the title 'hope.' That is how she feels moving forwards.

Clarissa has struggled with feelings of not being 'enough' for a long time. Before dancing the heart chakra, she took her wedding rings off for some reason and let them rest in jewellery cleaner while she danced. During her dance, she kept thinking of everyone else. She finally recognised that love towards herself was conspicuously absent. Afterwards, as she rested her left hand on the paper to create her mandala, she felt compelled to trace it. She realised that she didn't have her rings on. Inside the outline of her hand, she drew a heart—her heart—with wings on it. The message she took away was that, in order to grow and help others, she really needed to learn to love herself more and take better care of herself.

I encourage you to take a few moments to reflect on what you could do to be more kind and loving to yourself. Perhaps it's something simple like resting when you are tired, or taking more time for yourself when you need it. It may be eating more wholesome foods, or spending time with friends who are uplifting to be with. You may start noticing when you are judging or comparing yourself, and choose to accept and appreciate yourself more. If we set an intention to be kinder to ourselves, we will then be internally guided to what we most need.

Loving relationships

To thrive, we all need love in our lives. I don't necessarily mean the sentimental hearts and roses kind of love. I mean the love that's present in relationships when we are there for each other, even when things aren't pretty and beautiful.

It's in our nature to be loved and to love. We are not meant to journey through life alone. We need healthy connections which provide us with a sense of comfort and closeness—a shelter from the hard knocks of life.

I recently heard a story about some elephants who were going into towns, smashing and trampling on everything, before running away. Under normal circumstances, elephants don't behave like that. It was discovered that these particular elephants had all been taken away from their mothers and herds when they were young. They hadn't been loved or protected, and their destructive behaviour was a result of that.

As humans, we are much the same. If we don't have loving relationships in our lives, our natural way of being in the world gets distorted. We will feel deeply lonely and isolated, and may even behave in unloving ways. A key part of living a happy life is to experience the beauty and joy of true connection with others.

A simple way to bring more love into our lives is to start noticing when our family and friends need us. Love doesn't have to be about big grand gestures; we can show it in small ways. It may be helping your neighbour when you know she is struggling. Or giving your mum a call, when you know she's been at home on her own all day. Love is taking time out of your hectic schedule to really listen to your children when they are telling you about their day. It's about being attuned to the people around us, so that we know when we need to be there for them.

It can be challenging to stay in the energy of love, when those close to us are behaving in ways that irritate us. I recently watched an interview given by the author Brené Brown who said: *Assume that others are doing their best.* When we make this assumption, we're able to drop any judgements or blame and we naturally become more loving. I have found this simple statement to be such a gift. I encourage you to try it out in your relationships and see if it can help you become more loving in challenging circumstances.

We also need to be open to receiving love and kindness from others. So often we shrug off a compliment, or deny the help a friend is offering us. Opening up to love in our lives means receiving it with gratitude and grace. Open your heart to the hug your friend gives you. Breathe in any kind words. Accept the gift of love.

Time to try: *Cultivating Love*

Spend a few minutes each day directing the energy of kindness and gentleness to yourself, to any challenges you may be facing in your life, and to your relationships.

You can do this by breathing deeply and then imagining that your breath is filled with a rose pink light. This light is filled with love, kindness and gentleness. Breathe this light into your heart and, as you breathe out, direct the light to all the different parts of your body. You might start with your feet and slowly direct the light all the way up to your head. Imagine filling your whole body with love, kindness and gentleness.

Now allow any areas of difficulty, any challenges in your life, to gently drift into your mind. Breathe the pink light into your heart and, as you breathe out, imagine sending the light to these challenges. Spend as much time as you need sending love, kindness and compassion to any areas of your life that need it.

Finally, imagine a family member or friend sitting across from you. As you exhale, imagine sending the pink light of love and kindness to them. You may choose to focus on one person as you do this exercise, or you may send the light to a number of people in your life.

Sometimes it can be hard to allow yourself to receive love. Dancing the heart chakra, I felt as if little birds were unravelling stitches from my heart.

Kirsten

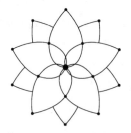

CHAPTER THIRTY-SEVEN

SHADOWS of the HEART

It's so easy to blame others when relationships go sour. Whether it's with a romantic partner or a friend, most of us are quick to judge and blame, seeing all of the wrong as being outside ourselves. In many cases, the relationship ends and we move on, only to discover that the same pattern shows up in our next relationship. Healing the heart chakra involves healing our own inner wounds and taking responsibility for the part we have played in our challenging relationships.

We have explored our shadow in the earlier chakras—the parts of ourselves that we have disowned and buried. One of the main ways we stay cut off from those parts of ourselves is by projecting them onto our relationships. We become convinced that the fault lies with our partner, failing to see the part we are playing.

For example, you may accuse your partner of being selfish, as he seems to do whatever he pleases without considering you or the family. You find his selfish behaviour drives you crazy, and you argue about it all the time. The level of hostility that this triggers in you, and the constant blaming, are indicators that there is something within you that you are projecting on to him. Hidden within, you may have a deep desire to escape and have your own adventures and freedom, but this desire feels selfish and wrong to you, and so you have buried it in your unconscious. You simply do not know that it is there. As you are unable to own this desire within yourself, you project it onto your partner, and you see it magnified as extreme selfishness in him. As you become more conscious of your hidden desires and take some steps to work with them (in this instance, something like planning a weekend escape with your girlfriends), the intensity of your reaction to your partner will fade.

We all project in our relationships, as we all have unconscious desires and wounds. The key is to see that our relationships are truly one of our greatest opportunities for our own growth, as they are like mirrors reflecting back to us what needs healing within ourselves. By working on owning our projections, we not only heal ourselves, but also bring harmony, maturity and genuine connection to our relationships.

The best way to begin working with projections is to reflect on what the huge trigger points are in your key relationships. They may be, for example, fidelity, laziness or control. Each time you are triggered, instead of lashing out, look within. Ask yourself what this issue is for you. Perhaps you have an attraction to a person outside of your relationship, but you may not have fully admitted this to yourself. You find yourself accusing your partner of being unfaithful, when really the desire to be unfaithful lies within you.

You may find your hidden wound showing up in many relationships. Perhaps you keep having romances that fizzle out quickly. At some deep level, you may feel unworthy of a partner who will stay with you, and so you keep attracting people into your life who reinforce this unconscious belief. To heal your relationship pattern, you need to heal the wound.

We unconsciously attract into our lives the exact relationships we need for our own healing. You may not know why you are drawn to a certain person, but something keeps bringing you back together. Trust that this will be the relationship that you need, in order to work through your deepest wounds. If both partners are committed to doing the work of withdrawing projections, the relationship can grow to a beautiful union of honesty, integrity and genuine love.

Meditation: *Healing Relationships*

This is a beautiful meditation that is done with the intention of bringing healing to our relationships and to ourselves.

You can do this meditation by reading the following steps, pausing after each one to imagine what has been described, or by listening to it with my voice-over guidance on the Heart Meditation Healing Relationship track: [refer to page vi]

1. Prepare your sacred space and yourself for your inner journey. Close your eyes and take three slow, deep breaths.

2. Imagine you are standing at the top of a large amphitheatre. You look across to the other side and see someone standing opposite. It is someone you currently have or have had a relationship with, and this relationship needs healing in some way. It may be a parent, child, partner, or even a part of you.

3. You look down into the centre of the amphitheatre and see a white lotus flower, gently curled into a bud. It has a magnificent light radiating from it. You are drawn to walk slowly down the stairs towards the light. With each step down, you take a full, deep breath. As you descend, the lotus flower opens wider and its light fills the whole space.

4. The person opposite you is stepping down into the light of the lotus in rhythm with you. You are looking into each other's eyes. After ten steps, you reach the centre of the flower, which is now pure light. You stand together, reaching out to hold both hands. You both breathe in the light. You are both bathed in healing light. Spend as much time here as you both need. Ask to be shown what it is in this relationship that reflects a need for healing within you. Be open to any insights, messages or feelings.

5. Now, have the intention to let go of the painful ties that are binding you. Watch them dissolve in the light, leaving only love.

6. Thank the person for what they have taught you, and then turn and walk slowly back up the stairs. As you reach the top, turn to look back. The other person is radiating light and you notice that you are too. The light from the amphitheatre lifts up into the sky and dissolves, transforming the pain you have left behind.

7. Take three deep breaths and bring your awareness back into your sacred space.

It's good to remember that the only person you can ever change in a relationship is you. This meditation will not change the behaviour of the other person. It will help you to heal your own wounds, which are showing up in this relationship. It will help you to release the painful ties. As you heal, the energy of the relationship will transform.

You may choose to return to this exercise several times. When you do, you may find different relationships, inner and outer, waiting for healing on the other side of the amphitheatre.

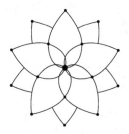

CHAPTER THIRTY-EIGHT

FORGIVING and LETTING GO

Throughout our lives, it is inevitable that we will get hurt in our relationships. Whether it is our relationship with our parents, partners, children or close friends, at some point we are bound to experience rejection, betrayal or loss of love. This is part of the human journey.

When we have been hurt, one of the most healing tools we have is the act of forgiveness. Forgiveness does not mean accepting that the hurtful behaviour of others was right or that we deserved it. Forgiveness is about choosing to let it go. When we do this, it can feel like we are letting someone get away with something, but the reality is that by not forgiving, we only hurt ourselves. When we choose to hold onto the hurt that someone has caused us, we shut down our own hearts.

Forgiving means releasing the block in our heart. We can forgive someone but still be cautious about trusting them again.

We can even forgive someone but still choose to end the relationship, because it doesn't serve us. Bringing in some healthy solar plexus boundaries is a wise move after forgiveness.

There is a French saying: *Tout comprendre c'est tout pardoner.* It means that to understand everything is to forgive everything. If we look closely at the people who cause us pain, we will typically find that they too are coming from a place of pain. I have found forgiveness to be easier when I choose to see beyond the behaviour to the real person inside.

As I was writing this chapter, a colleague I have been friends with for nearly ten years behaved in a way that I found very hurtful. My instant reaction was to want to attack back. I wrote an email in response, but I never sent it. As I read over what I had written, I could feel tightness in my chest. I realised that I was shutting down my heart chakra. It's often easier to resort to anger and retaliation than to sit with and feel the hurt.

Rather than send the email, I decided to dance the heart chakra. While I was dancing, I felt as though my friend was dancing with me. As we danced, I could feel her pain as well as mine. Feeling her pain helped me to understand why she had behaved the way she did. And in that moment I forgave her. I could feel a softening in my chest and a deepening of my breath as I did. Although it didn't change the situation, I felt like forgiveness was enough in this case. I am no longer carrying the hurt in my heart, so our relationship has been able to continue.

Forgiveness is not only about letting go of what others have done to us. It can also be about letting go of what we have done to hurt ourselves or others. Self-forgiveness can be even more challenging than forgiving others, because it requires us to take responsibility for our actions or thoughts, as well as let go of the negative feelings associated with them. Difficult though that may be, it's essential. If we continue to carry the burden in our hearts, we will never find freedom in our lives. Again, this is not about just letting ourselves off the hook. We need to feel the remorse, make amends, and learn from the experience. And then we need to release it.

When I was in my mid-twenties, I had a very close friend called Chris. Chris and I had worked together for a few years, and he had lived with my husband and me for nearly a year while he was househunting. One day, shortly after Chris had moved into his new house, he called me and asked if I would meet him for a drink that night. I was really stressed out with work and had a pounding headache, so I said no. Even though I could feel how much he desperately wanted me to meet him, I just couldn't face going out that night. The next day I found out that Chris had gone home that night and committed suicide.

For many years after, I held onto the torturous thought that if I had just met Chris for a drink that night and he had been able to share his problems with me, then he wouldn't have killed himself. I simply could not forgive myself. I could not let it go. I saw him in my dreams. I saw him in the faces of others on the street. I felt haunted by my decision.

One night, I decided to bring Chris into my dance of the heart chakra. I felt his presence with me and I wept and wept. I told him how sorry I was. I told him how much I missed him. And then I let him go. I let my decision not to meet him go too. I still think of Chris and I still wish I had met him for a drink that night, but it no longer haunts me in the same way. I chose to forgive myself and release the pain I was carrying.

Time to try: *A Forgiveness Prayer*

A few years ago, I was invited to be part of a women's healing circle. We met regularly to meditate, dance and share stories. At one of our meetings, a woman led us through a beautiful prayer of forgiveness, which was based on Ho'oponopono, the Hawaiian practice of forgiveness. The prayer is simple: *I am sorry. Please forgive me. I love you. Thank you.*

Here is a self-practice that evolved out of the above experience, where you quietly say or sing the prayer. Begin with *I'm sorry*, which may be directed at you in response to some kind of pain you have caused yourself, like abusing your body or thinking unkind thoughts about yourself. Or your *I'm sorry* may be directed at someone else, because of the way you treated that person. Bring the situation into your mind and then really feel your *I'm sorry*. Then repeat the rest of the prayer, committing fully to the intention inherent in the words: *I am sorry. Please forgive me. I love you. Thank you.*

When I practised this prayer, I found myself crying unexpectedly. I could physically feel the tension in my heart release. I could feel a softening taking place. It really helped me to feel just how powerful forgiveness is, if we can genuinely do it.

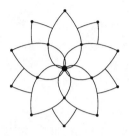

CHAPTER THIRTY-NINE

the COMPASSIONATE HEART

The heart harbours a great paradox. When we go through the complete healing process of surrendering into our pain, sitting in the darkness of our grief, and then finally letting it all go, we are rewarded with treasure at the end. This treasure is an expanded heart capable of deeper levels of compassion.

There is a Sufi prayer that says: *Shatter my heart, so a new room can be created for a Limitless Love.* It's as though our own journey through the dark night of the soul opens us to a deeper understanding of humanity. Experiencing the loss or pain of personal love somehow cracks us open, to the point where we are able to find deep compassion for others and the pain they are facing. We experience a more profound, sacred love. We are able to walk our path with heart.

Walking with heart means walking through life with loving kindness and generosity. There is a return to a childlike state, when we peel back the layers and open ourselves up to a limitless love. Our world can feel so harsh, and it is often small gestures that can cause great shifts—within others but also within ourselves.

I remember taking my daughter into the city of Sydney for a shopping trip. She was about five years old and she needed new shoes. As we leapt off the bus and headed towards the department store, we noticed a beggar on the side of the road. Hundreds of people were rushing past the beggar, pretending not to see her. This lady was mute and had made a sign to explain her situation. My little daughter tried to read the sign, but needed help. As I read the lady's message out loud, it became very difficult to do what everyone else was doing and simply ignore the feelings she was bringing out in me.

As the lady locked eyes with mine, I felt something happen. I saw the light in her eyes and I felt her light in my heart. By this gentle human connection, we were both touched in some way. My daughter decided that she wanted to give the lady the money we were going to spend on shoes, and so we did. We silently thanked each other, and my daughter and I began our walk back to the bus stop. In many ways, I feel I received more from the mute lady than she did from me that day.

There is a softening that happens when we come home to our hearts. Through our vulnerability, we open to a deeper intelligence—a heart-based intelligence. We find natural empathy and compassion for fellow human beings. We treat the animal kingdom and our planet with respect. You only need to look at what is going on in the world to see that there is a collective shadow in the world's heart that needs healing. Only when enough people rise into the sacred love of the heart will we see a reflection of this in the world around us.

Love is really all there is. If we could all live from an open heart, the world would be a very different place. Love is such a healing force. Although gentle, it can dissolve the most intense pain.

Mother Teresa comes to mind, as I write about the healing power of love. She showed us how gentleness and kindness can be so deeply transforming to so many. Her work helped the poor, the dying, orphans, lepers and AIDS sufferers. We don't all need to start charities, but we can channel the energy of Mother Teresa in our everyday lives. Who do you know who is feeling poor, sick or orphaned on the inside?

Mother Teresa once said: *The greatest disease in the West today is not TB or leprosy; it is being unwanted, unloved and uncared for. We can cure physical diseases with medicine, but the only cure for loneliness, despair and hopelessness is love. There are many in the world who are dying for a piece of bread, but there are many more dying for a little love. The poverty in the West is a different kind of poverty—it is not only a poverty of loneliness but also of spirituality. There's a hunger for love, as there is a hunger for God.*

One of the most powerful ways of giving love is to simply be there for someone with an open heart, to hold 'heart space' for them. Holding heart space means being there for someone through whatever journey they are on. We don't judge them or try to fix them. We don't make them feel inadequate or tell them what we think they should do. We don't try to control them or their situation in any way. We simply walk alongside them offering gentle support. The person we are holding space for can then be vulnerable, without fear of judgement. They can feel safe. This is unconditional love. This is compassion. Holding heart space for someone is a way of saying, 'I see you. And I'm here for you.'

The Sanskrit word *namaste* is used as a respectful greeting in India, Nepal and other parts of Asia. *Namaste* represents the belief that there is a divine spark of light within each of us. As we say *namaste*, we place our hands together in the prayer position at our heart chakra, to connect with divine love. Then we softly bow our heads in respect. When we greet someone with the *namaste* gesture, it is like the light of our soul is acknowledging the soul light of that person.

This is such a beautiful example of how we can greet every being we encounter during our day. Even when people behave in ways we don't like, relating to them from this point of acknowledgment has to have an impact at some level. When we respect ourselves and we respect others, energy shifts. This is living life from an open heart.

Moving into the heart chakra often compels us to want to help those less fortunate than ourselves. We might be called to help refugees, the homeless, or those suffering from domestic violence. If you feel a natural calling to a particular need, follow it. I feel that our heart is like our compass: it guides us to where we need to go.

The Dalai Lama said: *Love and compassion are necessities, not luxuries. Without them humanity cannot survive.* Trust the calling of your heart—the world needs it.

Time to try: *Heart Wishes*

Heart Wishes is a simple, yet deeply powerful practice to incorporate into our daily lives. It only takes a few minutes, and it helps to open our compassionate heart:

1. For this exercise you will need a candle—a small tea light is enough. Light the candle and let your gaze rest softly on the flickering light. Tune into the natural rhythm of your breathing and connect with your heart chakra.
2. Begin by making a wish for yourself. Your wish may be to find more peace and love in your life. It may be to find forgiveness.

Let your wish come from your heart space, rather than your head.

3. Next, make a wish for a loved one.
4. Finally, make a wish for someone you may be in conflict with.
5. To finish, blow out the candle and send the light to your wishes.

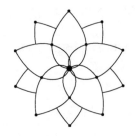

CHAPTER FORTY

DANCING the HEART CHAKRA

Dancing the heart chakra was more of a gentle release than I'd imagined. I found the music beautiful, which allowed a real heart connection. There were moments I felt a welling up of emotion. As I allowed my tears to fall, my heart told me to rejoice. I then danced as a leaf being carried up by the wind, talking with the treetops. I felt energetic golden threads connecting me to the beauty and love of all that is. This dance felt very precious and tender.

Jessica

It is now time to move your heart chakra. Create your sacred space and prepare yourself for the dance. Take a few minutes to breathe deeply into your heart chakra at the centre of your chest.

You may even want to cup your hands gently over your heart chakra and feel the warmth from your hands pour into your heart.

When you are ready, play the Move Your Heart Chakra music [refer to page vi] and feel the vibration of the crystal bowl pulsing at your heart chakra. Close your eyes and let go. Feel yourself being lifted by the joyful, expansive music.

The music may call you to open and expand your chest, creating a softening of your heart. You may feel like you are becoming lighter, even weightless. Exaggerate your breath, to create movement in your body. Physically express the in and out, the giving and receiving, with your hands and arms. Imagine inhaling love and exhaling peace in your dance. As you embody the healing energies of love, joy and compassion, any excess energy held within your heart can begin to release.

Once you have finished your dance, take three slow, deep breaths, then sit down to create your mandala art.

I loved the music and, as I danced, I could see all these spirits around me, dancing with me. One of these spirits was that of a close friend who had committed suicide. She was dancing with me, and I could see she was really happy. Somehow dancing the heart chakra healed the grief of losing my friend, and I was able to let go of her, and of the pain around that situation.

Amanda

Chanting the heart chakra

The mantra sound for the heart chakra is YAM, which is pronounced as YUM. Try chanting this sound to help balance your heart chakra.

Sit peacefully and bring your awareness to your breathing. Inhale fully through your nose. As you exhale, vocalise the mantra YAM while focusing your awareness at the centre of your chest. I recommend chanting for around five minutes, or however long feels right for you.

Take notice of any feelings, memories, images or sensations that come up for you as you chant. Spend a few minutes coming back to your natural breathing to finish.

For more information on chanting the chakras, please see Chapter 44: Sacred Singing and Chanting.

Heart chakra affirmation: *I am loved.*
I am at peace. My heart is open.

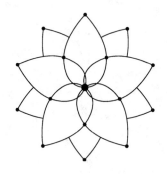

PART 7

MOVING YOUR
THROAT CHAKRA

*I found the throat chakra to be the most
powerful dance of them all.
I had suppressed myself, my voice and my creativity for a
very long time. I was the kind of person who had never sung
in front of people, and I didn't speak up for myself. When
I got to the throat chakra, I experienced a lot of throat
clearing—literally feeling like it was very gluggy, full of debris.
I almost felt like I was suffocating, so I started clearing and
clearing my throat. Gradually I could feel it becoming free.
Then I began to purr, and as I purred like a lion,
I realised my throat felt like it was expanding.
Because of my throat chakra clearing, I've
blossomed, creatively and personally.*

Cynthia

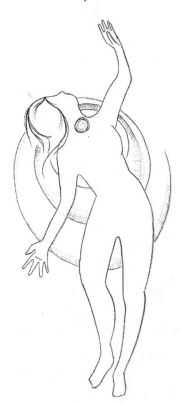

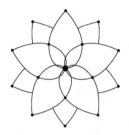

CHAPTER FORTY-ONE

AUTHENTIC EXPRESSION

The throat chakra is our source of communication. When it is balanced, we are able to express ourselves freely, authentically and creatively. We are able to live according to our own truth. It's as though we sing the song of our soul out into the world.

Sadly for so many of us, our life experiences can cause us to shut down our authentic expression. We learn to hide who we truly are. We wear different masks when we interact with others, in an attempt to shield ourselves from the world.

When I was studying psychology, I came across the work of a psychoanalyst named Donald Winnicott. He is known for his ideas on what he calls 'the true self' and 'the false self,' which describe different functions of our psychology. As soon as I began studying his theories, they immediately resonated with me. He described the true self as our authentic self, the part of us that is the source of our creativity and spontaneity. When we are connected to our true self, we feel genuinely alive inside and are able to express ourselves naturally and freely. He believed that our true self begins developing when we are young children. When our parents or primary caregivers respond in reassuring ways to our feelings and expressions, we learn that nothing bad will happen when we are being real. So there is no need to try to control who we are, or pretend to be someone else. We learn to be real and express ourselves authentically.

By contrast, the false self starts to develop when we are young, if our environment feels unsafe or overwhelming or if we have to put on a mask to comply with the expectations of others. Rather than spontaneously expressing our own feelings and ideas, we learn to anticipate others' demands and comply with them, as a way of protecting our true self from a world that feels unsafe. Unfortunately, if we keep these masks on as we grow up, we start to believe that this false self is who we really are. Even if we go on to have successful lives, there is always a sense of numbness inside. We are not genuinely happy, because part of us is living in hiding, often without us even knowing it.

Part of healing the throat chakra is about reconnecting with our true self and finding our freedom of expression. This involves peeling off our masks and revealing who we truly are inside. According to Marion Woodman, one of my favourite Jungian authors: *If we have lived our lives behind a mask, sooner or later—if we are lucky—that mask will be smashed.*

Silvia felt as though she had spent a lot of her life wearing a mask and pretending to be someone else. She began to realise just how exhausting it was to live that way, especially as she wasn't able to satisfy everybody anyway, no matter how much she pretended. Her life looked perfect from the outside, but inside she felt a deep sense of emptiness and inexplicable sadness.

The more Silvia danced the throat chakra, the more she started to realise that it was time to stop being so afraid of showing who she really was. She received a clear message of 'no more masks, no more roles, no more merciful lies and excuses.' She decided it was time to express how she really felt and what she really wanted. She realised that sometimes we need to give up the perfect life, in order to have a real one.

Living from a place of truth can feel vulnerable at times. But ultimately, it is very freeing. In the early days of my Chakradance practice, whenever I danced the throat chakra I would see an image of a beautiful, bright blue bird stuck in a cage. The bird would fly wildly around the cage, trying to spread its wings and find freedom, but it was trapped. At this time in my life, I felt very uncomfortable being my authentic self around a lot of people. My family thought that the world of chakras and energy work was all a bit weird and 'woo woo.' I worked during the day in the competitive industry of advertising recruitment, so I spent a lot of time hiding parts of myself. As time moved on, that bright blue bird in the cage became more and more desperate. It needed to get out.

There comes a time in our lives when, if we are going to be free, we have to reveal who we really are. Taking off our mask can feel like coming out of the closet. There is a chance that we are going to be rejected, criticised and judged. Yet, even if that happens, we will discover that the freedom that comes from being real is far more powerful than worrying about what others might think of us.

When I finally let the blue bird out of the cage, my life began to transform. I stepped fully into my Chakradance career and began sharing it with others. I wrote a book about it. I talked about it on TV. I flew to the other side of the world to run large groups. I began to sing the song of my soul out into the world. This was a huge healing for me, as there had been a lot of fear around showing who I really was.

I now accept that not everyone will resonate with my expression, and I know that that's okay. The more we live our lives in alignment with who we truly are, the more comfortable we become with not having to be understood by everyone. The added beauty is that we are more easily able to accept others for who they truly are. What I've also found is that the more authentic we are, the more we begin to attract into our lives the people and opportunities that do naturally resonate with us.

As I danced the throat chakra, a huge wave of sorrow came over me and I found myself crying. I saw myself (or my soul) shackled with something that looked like barbed wire and I was trying to shake it off. My soul struggled to express itself freely. Its message to me was: 'Be Yourself.'

Silvia

When I danced the throat chakra, I felt like I was connecting with something familiar. It was a feeling of recognising something within myself that had been hidden. It felt like I was releasing some kind of fear. I felt quite emotional. I felt like I was seeing an old friend again.

Natalie

Meditation: *Meeting Your Hidden Self*

When we lose touch with our true self, the throat chakra can be like a gateway back to that inner energy. This meditation is designed to lead us on a gentle journey within, to bring healing to the parts of us that may have been buried, hurt or scared in the past.

In this meditation, you may reunite with parts of yourself that you know are hiding, and you may also discover some unknown aspects of yourself. I suggest trying it several times, because you may connect with different parts of yourself each time you do it.

You can do this meditation by reading the following steps, pausing after each one to imagine what has been described, or by listening to it with my voice-over guidance on the Throat Chakra Meditation: Meeting Your Hidden Self track: [refer to page vi]

1. Prepare your sacred space and yourself. Softly close your eyes, and take three slow, deep breaths.

2. Imagine you are stepping through a curtain of sheer white fabric. It feels like you are stepping through a veil into another world. It's like being inside a beautiful crystal chamber. Everything is shimmering and sparkling, and you can hear the sounds of gentle harmonies. It feels very safe and magical.

3. As you step further inside, you see that there are hundreds of beautiful blue butterflies. The butterflies all take flight together and slowly move towards you. Then they gently fly off together, inviting you to follow them. Intrigued, you follow the butterflies and see that they are leading you to a circle made of crystals.

4. As you get closer, you can see that a person is sitting in the circle. The butterflies lead you to the centre of the circle, and you find yourself sitting opposite the person, looking into her eyes. As you gaze into those familiar eyes, the butterflies begin flying around the crystals, creating a gentle vortex of blue. You feel safe and held.

5. As you sit with this person, you know that she is a part of you. She has been hiding here in this safe circle, waiting for the day when you would be ready to come and find her. She has had times in her life when she didn't feel safe, when she

felt hurt or scared. As you spend time with her, do whatever feels right to reassure her that she is safe and loved. You may wish to hold hands or hug her. There may be things she wants to tell you. Spend as much time as you need here.

6. After some time, the blue butterflies fly into the centre of the circle and begin moving so quickly that it feels like you are both sitting in the centre of a blue flame. It feels like a fire, but it has no heat. The blue flame is transmuting any painful experiences. As the flame dances around you and through you, you see the person in front of you transforming into you. You close your eyes and breathe in the blue healing energy, knowing that you are together once again.

7. The blue butterflies lead you back through the crystal chamber and you gently step back through the sheer white veil, returning to your everyday life.

8. Take three slow, deep breaths and bring your awareness back into your space.

You may feel emotional after this meditation. If you do, spend some time sitting in your sacred space and breathing gently. I would also encourage you to journal about your experience, or find a symbolic way to acknowledge what has taken place.

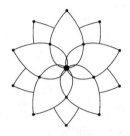

CHAPTER FORTY-TWO

CREATIVE EXPRESSION

One of the keys to rediscovering and expressing our true self is our creativity. We are all creative beings, whether we know it or not. So many people I work with tell me they have no creativity. It always makes me smile, because they then express themselves wildly through their own free dance or mandala art making.

Many of us have preconceived ideas about what creativity is. A beautiful looking painting? A song with perfect harmonies? This is not the kind of creativity we need to rediscover to find freedom in our lives. The creativity we need is not about perfection, or even about the end product. It's about the raw, truthful expression of what's really inside us. When we connect with this creativity, it becomes a healing force.

I see our creativity as being like a double gateway. It can lead us into our inner world, helping us reach the depths of who are, but it can also express these inner parts of us in the outer world, revealing back to us what we have previously been unable to see. With true creativity, we go in, we surrender, we feel, we hurt—we go fully into chaos, to find our hidden selves. Genuine creativity isn't always pretty. Quite often it's an expression of the pain we have buried inside or the unknown shadow within us.

I know that whenever I surrender into dance, I find truth. I may not always like what comes, but it's always truth that I both find and express.

When I was studying psychology, I became good friends with a fellow student who was a painter. After she had spent months painting for her next exhibition, I went along to support her on opening night. As I strolled around the gallery, I started to get a sinking feeling in my stomach. She had painted many female nudes, and most of them had some kind of wound in the right breast. Her art, combined with some dreams I knew she was having, indicated to me that her unconscious was desperately trying to communicate with her. It turned out that she had breast cancer and, for months, her unconscious had been sending her signals through her art. The fact that her art revealed her cancer to her—long before she could feel it in her body—shows how powerful our creative expression is. In such cases, it can even save our lives.

There are so many forms of creative expression. If you haven't found yours yet, then experiment. It could be painting, sculpture, photography, playing music, singing, dancing, chanting, or even drawing in the dirt. What makes you feel? What brings your buried tears to the surface? What transports you to places of unbelievable beauty?

Giri grew up being told that she didn't have a creative bone in her body. There was a time, not that long ago, when had a circle been put in front of her and she'd been asked to draw something inside it, she would have just sat there and cried. Since practising the dance of the throat chakra, her creativity has started to flow.

She is now expressing herself through her choice of clothing, her cooking, and even through public speaking.

Many of us are like Giri. We have been told that we are not creative, or we have become caught up in what the finished product will be like, so we censor our expression. Healing the throat chakra removes those obstacles, so that our genuine creative expression can flow naturally.

Time to try: *Morning Pages*

Many years ago, I came across an amazing book on how to rediscover our creativity. It's called *The Artist's Way* by Julia Cameron. Julia shares lots of different methods for unlocking creativity, and one of the exercises that I have personally done for many years is called Morning Pages.

In this exercise, upon waking in the morning, you immediately put pen to paper and write three pages in longhand. The idea is that you don't let your pen stop moving. You don't censor your expression and you don't think about what you are writing. It's pure stream of consciousness. If you can't think of anything to say, you might write: 'I can't think of anything to say.' Nothing is too ridiculous. It is important that the morning pages are done every day. The other key is knowing that no-one will ever read them except you, so you have complete freedom to let go.

The morning pages achieve a number of things. First, they release all the noise—the chaotic thoughts and dramas in our minds that block us from our creativity. Julia describes the reason for doing morning pages as: *To get to the other side ... the other side of our fear, our negativity, our moods ... and our censor.* Writing these pages is almost like a meditation, where we clear a path through the chaos, in order to reach a different space within us.

Secondly, the morning pages plant the seed of creativity within us. Having done morning pages religiously for a number of years, I've found that among all the crazy, silly and pathetic stuff that I wrote were the seeds of creative ideas. I found truths that I hadn't known, until they came pouring out. My morning pages became peppered with inspiration for my creativity.

If you are truly looking to unlock your creativity, I highly recommend writing your morning pages every day, as well as regularly dancing your throat chakra.

Dancing the throat chakra has really helped
me experience and express my creativity.
I've started writing and painting.

Cynthia

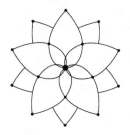

CHAPTER FORTY-THREE

VERBAL EXPRESSION

We communicate all the time, but how much of what we say is truthful and authentic? How many times have we said 'yes' when we really wanted to say 'no'? How often have we found ourselves swallowing the words we would really like to say? When we don't speak our truth, our communication is incongruent; our words say one thing, while our body language and energy say something completely different. Balancing the throat chakra leads us to a place where we can be authentic in the way we communicate, where we can find resonance between our words and our truth.

This resonance is so important, because words are not intangible or ephemeral—they carry vibrations. Just think of a time when you were with friends or family and everyone was talking, but there was no meaningful conversation going on. It was all chitchatting, gossiping or complaining about things. We typically come away from those types of conversations feeling drained. The vibrations of the words have literally dragged us down.

Now think of a time when someone said something hurtful to or about you. That old saying: *Sticks and stones may break my bones but names will never hurt me* is not true. Words can feel like a physical blow. After all, singers can break glass with their voice alone. Harsh words can be just as damaging.

Many years ago, I saw a film called *What the Bleep Do We Know?*. It was based on the experiments of Dr. Masaru Emoto, who wanted to find out what kind of physical effect words, prayer and music would have on the structure of water. In one experiment, he exposed water to words, then froze it into crystalline structures and photographed the results. The findings were incredible. The water that had been exposed to positive words was symmetrical and beautiful. The water that had been exposed to negative words was jagged and unattractive. Human beings are made up of sixty percent water, so you can imagine how we are affected by words and how our words affect others.

Have you ever listened to a motivational speaker or spiritual leader whose words were transforming? When we experience such a moment, we come away feeling more positive and energised. The vibrations of such words can literally shift our energy.

We all have the opportunity to lift the vibrational frequency of our words. Healing the throat chakra helps us to become more mindful of the type of communication we want to engage in. We begin to notice how much more alive we feel when we are speaking truthfully and with integrity. We feel uplifted when we speak positively and have meaningful conversations with others.

Several years ago I attended a Buddhist meditation retreat, where I learnt about the Buddhist precept of 'wise speech'. To practise wise speech, we ask ourselves four questions before we engage in an important conversation: *Is it true? Is it kind? Is it necessary? Is it the right time?* Learning this was hugely powerful for me.

It's so easy to get caught up in a heated discussion with someone and speak from a place of pain, anger or unconsciousness. When this happens, we are often left feeling deflated and regretful about some of the things we have said. Filtering our conversation through the precept of wise speech can dramatically change our communications for the better. What we say becomes more conscious and more considered. We lift the vibrational frequency of our words.

When Edie found Chakradance, she had been estranged from her mother for many, many years. She had every reason never to speak to her mother again, given what had happened during her childhood. By dancing the heart chakra, Edie had found some forgiveness for her mother. However, it was her work on her throat chakra and her communication skills that really helped bring healing to their relationship.

A few months into her Chakradance practice, Edie's mother called to talk. Instead of rushing to get off the phone, Edie found herself having a real and honest conversation. She managed to share with her mother how she had felt for so long and she did it from a loving and kind place. She couldn't believe how easily she was able to communicate the pain and suffering she had been through, without blaming her mother or falling apart. They talked for hours that day and Edie knew that her mother could truly hear her. Her mother apologised for hurting her and for failing her. It felt like a true miracle. They now have lots of talks that are filled with laughter and love.

Self-talk

In addition to communicating with others, we are always communicating with ourselves. There is a powerful quote by the Sufi poet Hafiz that says: *The words you speak become the house you live in.* When I first heard those words, I couldn't help but think about how little regard so many of us have, not only for the words we speak to others, but also for the constant inner dialogue we have with ourselves.

How often do you catch yourself saying something negative to yourself? *I'm not good enough. I can't do that. I'm not smart enough. I'm not pretty enough.* Most of us have a negative internal dialogue happening on a semi-regular basis. Sometimes it's other people's words that we have internalised; sometimes we are just speaking harshly to ourselves. If our words are creating our reality, we need to take responsibility for what we are saying to ourselves.

A powerful way of healing the throat chakra is through positive affirmations. The late inspirational author and teacher, Louise Hay, was famous for this kind of work. She used affirmations to heal herself from cancer, then went on to help millions of people transform their lives. Affirmations work best when they are said in the present tense. They need to be positive, personal and specific. We speak them aloud, frequently and with conviction, in our own unique voice. What do you need to affirm to yourself?

We can create affirmations for different areas of our lives. I like to create affirmations for each of the chakras. Here is a simple example of an affirmation for each:

- Base chakra: *I love every part of my body. Every cell is filled with energy and vitality.*
- Sacral chakra: *I am sensual and passionate. My sexual energy is sacred.*
- Solar plexus chakra: *I am worthy. I am powerful. I courageously follow my own unique path.*
- Heart chakra: *I am loved. I am at peace. My heart is open.*
- Throat chakra: *I live an authentic life. I speak my truth.*
- Third eye chakra: *I trust my intuition. I see clearly.*

- Crown chakra: *I am connected to and supported by everything in the Universe.*

Feel free to try these affirmations or create your own.

Time to try: *The Humming Breath*

Another powerful way of using the positive vibration of words is through this humming breath exercise. It can be done while sitting or standing, even while in the shower. I often bring the humming breath into my dance of the throat chakra:

1. Begin by gently pulling your shoulders back, so that your spine is straight. Softly close your eyes.
2. Bring your awareness to your breath, as you breathe in through your nose and out through your mouth. After a minute or so, exhale and make a soft humming sound like a bee. Pause as you breathe in, and then continue to hum as you breathe out. Continue with this humming breath for a few minutes, feeling the vibration in your throat.
3. Reflect on a word that holds the vibration you most need in your life right now. It may be love, peace, joy or something else. Take a deep breath in through your nose and sound out the word as you exhale. Feel the vibration of this word. Send this vibration through and around your whole body. Repeat as many times as feels right for you.
4. Now choose a word that holds the vibration you would most like to send to a particular person or to a place in the world that needs healing. As you exhale, have the intention of sending this vibration out to the person or place.
5. Finish by returning to normal breathing and slowly open your eyes.

Practising the humming breath exercise helps us to feel the different vibrations of each of the words we choose to sound. It helps us to respect the power of our words and how they impact on us and on the world around us.

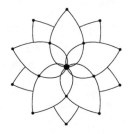

CHAPTER FORTY-FOUR

SACRED SINGING
and CHANTING

Taking the humming breath one step further, we can use the healing vibrations of sacred singing and chanting as a beautiful way of communicating. Throughout my life, I have been moved by many experiences of sacred singing. My family are Catholic, and I went to church every Sunday morning as a child. I loved the sense of ritual that came with being at church, but mostly I loved the singing of the hymns. Although I couldn't understand why at the time, singing hymns always lifted my energy and left me feeling happier and more at peace. Now I know that the combination of ritual and sacred singing is really a form of vibrational and spiritual healing.

When my daughter was five, we decided to join a choir in Sydney. We were looking for a creative activity we could do together, and joined the Threshold Choir. Each week we would sit in a circle as a group and we would sing beautiful lullabies, gentle hymns and prayers. At the end of each class, a chair that looked a bit like a sun lounge would be put in the middle of the circle, and we would take turns lying on the chair while the group sang to us. My daughter and I would lie there together and receive these beautiful sounds. It felt like being caressed, like being held by sound. We would always leave feeling so calm and peaceful.

Afterwards, many members of the choir would go out to hospitals and homes and sing to people in the final hours of their lives. They became sacred instruments to help those on the threshold of dying. One of the women described it as kindness and peace made audible. The power of voice—our words, our sounds and our vibrations—has never been shown more clearly to me than by this choir.

More recently, a friend introduced me to the age-old practice of chanting mantras. Mantras are the sacred sounds of Sanskrit, the ancient language of India. When we chant mantras, we evoke a specific vibration and open up to the sacred wisdom contained in each sound.

Each chakra has a specific mantra sound. These sounds are called *bija* in Sanskrit (seed sounds). When we chant a seed sound, it feels like an activation—a gateway leading us deep into that chakra. When I chant the mantras for the chakras, I often see a beautiful, ornate wooden door with a large keyhole. It's as though the sound becomes the key and the door unlocks and opens. The vibration of the sound then leads me into the dwelling of whatever chakra I am chanting. Any feelings, images, sensations or memories that surface are directly related to that chakra.

When we chant a *bija* sound, we connect with our own personal chakra. But something else happens too. Millions of people have chanted the same sacred sound for thousands of years so when we chant, it can feel like we are not chanting alone. We are tapping into a collective experience and merging with a greater consciousness. There is a profound feeling of being connected to the greater rhythm of life.

Time to try: *Chanting Chakra Sounds*

Try chanting the sacred sound for each chakra. Start by sitting peacefully, bringing your awareness to your breathing. Inhale fully through your nose. As you exhale, vocalise the mantra of each chakra, one at a time. Try focusing your attention on the physical location of each chakra as you chant its sound, then feel the vibration expand throughout your whole body and beyond. Chant each chakra as many times as feels comfortable for you.

Chakra	Location	Sound
Base	Perineum area	LAM (pronounced LUM)
Sacral	Above pubic bone	VAM (pronounced VUM)
Solar plexus	Above navel	RAM (pronounced RUM)
Heart	Chest area	YAM (pronounced YUM)
Throat	Throat area	HAM (pronounced HUM)
Third eye	Between eyebrows	OM (pronounced AUM)
Crown	Top of head	Silence or Nngg (as in sing)

Take notice of any feelings, memories, images or sensations that come up for you as you chant. Spend a few minutes coming back to your natural breathing to finish.

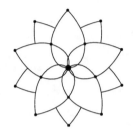

CHAPTER FORTY-FIVE

LISTENING and the GIFT of BEING HEARD

The other vital aspect of communication is listening. As we balance our throat chakra, we open up to a much deeper level of listening. It's not just about hearing people's words. We pick up on the tone of their voice, their body language, and the emotion behind what they are saying. We may even notice when they are holding back their words.

We are vibrational beings and we listen not just with our ears, but with our whole being. The more balanced our throat chakra, the more highly attuned our listening skills are.

One of the most profound human needs is to be heard. When someone deeply listens to us, this basic need is met. Even if there is no change to our circumstances, just having someone fully hear our story and our feelings brings about a healing. Being heard validates our truth and helps us to move forwards.

Sadly, many of us have grown up without being truly heard. This is something that comes up frequently when we reach the throat chakra in Chakradance.

When Leslie danced the throat chakra, she connected with the part of her that felt like a silenced child. Leslie grew up in a large family who were always fighting. She was painfully shy and used to hide up in the trees just to be alone. Physically, she suffered with strep throat for many years. She now has a raging ex-husband; her main issue with her current husband is that he just doesn't listen to her. Dancing the throat chakra wasn't easy for her. She kept forgetting to breathe. As Leslie chanted with the music, she sounded like a child with a squeaky voice. The more she danced, the more she could remember all the instances when she had not been heard, had not been understood. She could see how this had caused her to hide and not speak her truth. The message she received from her silenced child was: 'It's time to speak up. It's time to be heard.'

Deep listening is vital to balancing the throat chakra, which means listening to others, as well as listening to our own inner voice. There is often so much chatter going on inside us that it can be challenging to hear what our authentic voice is saying.

When I attended a Buddhist meditation retreat, I spent ten days in silence. We weren't allowed to communicate with anyone. We weren't even allowed any eye contact. Also, we weren't allowed any external stimulus—no reading or writing. We spent our time sitting and focusing on our breathing. That was when I began to realise how much internal noise was covering up my true voice. I found myself having future conversations with people in my head. Then I would be back in the past, saying something that I wished I had said back then. I flitted backwards and forwards in time, internally chattering all the way. It was exhausting and confusing.

After several days of silence, meditation and no distractions, I began to catch myself having these pointless conversations. I would gently let them go and return to my breath. At some point, I began to hear a different voice. This voice came from a deeper place and held a deeper vibration. It held the vibration of truth, the vibration of wisdom. The messages were simple but very clear. I learnt that this voice can only be heard when we are fully present and when we have opened ourselves to deep inner listening.

You may have heard of the term 'clairaudience.' Many psychics use this term to define what they do. Clairaudience simply means clear hearing. When our throat chakra is open, we hear not only our own inner guidance, but also the guidance of higher realms. This is not a supernatural power; this is something that is genuinely available to all of us, as we clear our throat chakras.

In addition to dancing the throat chakra, I recommend spending some sustained periods in silence. I know that this can be challenging to organise for many of us. But committing to just fifteen minutes of silence a day can have a profound impact on what we hear from our internal world.

Listening, hearing, speaking my truth and being heard. A hive of bees infused me until I became a prayer—my dance of the throat chakra.

Carol

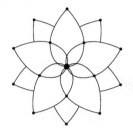

CHAPTER FORTY-SIX

HOW SOUNDS AFFECT US

The sounds we hear from the outer world also impact on our throat chakras. Many of us are bombarded with noise so much of the time. Just take a moment and listen now. What can you hear? There are usually constant noises from the outside world—traffic, electronics, people talking. We spend so much time and energy unconsciously trying to tune out the discordant sounds around us.

Balancing the throat chakra calls us to take responsibility for the sounds we invite in. We can't always control the uninvited sounds around us, but we can choose to bring more harmonious sounds into our lives. We can choose to play beautiful music and feel it touching us. We can sit by the ocean and let the sound of the waves wash through us. Sounds and their vibrations can be healing or harmful. Balancing the throat chakra involves making a commitment to bring more healing sounds into our lives.

Spend some time reflecting on the sounds in your daily life. Where can you make healthy changes? For example, turn off the television unless you are actively watching it. Put on peaceful music while you are making dinner. Turn humming electronics off when you are sleeping. Small changes such as these can make a big difference to the health of our throat chakra.

Time to try: *Sound Check*

Quite often we are unaware of all of the sounds impacting on us, day in and day out. A great way to gain some awareness is to choose a day, then use your journal to record all the sounds you hear throughout it. Pay particular attention to the first sounds you hear when you wake up, because these sounds set the mood for your whole day. Is your alarm clock literally alarming you every morning? What sounds do you hear as you travel to work? What sounds are you taking in as you eat your lunch?

At the end of the day, go through your list of sounds and notice how many are healing and how many are harming. Reflect on how you could minimise unhealthy sounds and maximise healthy ones. For example, you may need to get a new alarm clock with a more soothing sound to wake up to. You may choose to wear headphones and listen to beautiful music as you sit on a noisy train. You may invest in a water feature, so you can hear the trickling of water instead of your chatty neighbours as you eat lunch on the verandah.

Think of it as if you are creating the soundtrack for your daily life. What music do you want to dance your life to?

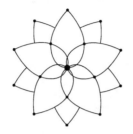

CHAPTER FORTY-SEVEN

DANCING the
THROAT CHAKRA

*As I danced the throat chakra, I felt vibrational healing
emanating from my throat, chest and the palms of my
hands. I felt the mantra vibrating through my whole
body and I felt surrounded by crystalline shafts of
vibrational white light. I could feel the power I have to
heal myself and others by simply speaking divine truth.*

Gilly

It is now time to move your throat chakra. Create your sacred
space and prepare yourself for your dance.

The dance of the throat chakra is a mantra dance, where we
chant ourselves into dance. Begin by taking a few deep breaths.
Exaggerate the sound of your outbreath. Gently chant the sound
HAM (pronounced HUM), to activate your throat chakra. Feel
the tingling sensation in your throat, as it vibrates with sound.

When you are ready, play the Move Your Throat music [refer to page vi] and feel the vibration of the crystal bowl resonating at your throat chakra. Close your eyes and surrender into your own mantra dance.

You may want to continue chanting the mantra of HAM throughout your dance, or chant a word with the vibration you would most like to have pulsing through your body (like love or peace). You may find that other sounds just naturally begin to pour out of you. By surrendering to the music, you will find yourself dancing from the inside out. You will find movements and sounds that express your inner truth. As you dance the throat chakra, it may feel as though you are harmonising in a ceremony of sacred sounds. It can feel like dancing with the greater rhythm of life.

Once you have finished your dance, take three slow, deep breaths, then sit down to create your mandala art.

Chanting the Throat Chakra

You may like to spend a few minutes focusing specifically on chanting the mantra sound for the throat chakra, which is HAM (pronounced as HUM). Relax and bring your awareness to your breathing. Inhale fully through your nose. As you exhale, vocalise the mantra HAM while focusing your awareness at your throat. Be mindful of any feelings, memories, images or sensations that come up for you as you chant. Spend a few minutes coming back to your natural breathing to finish.

Throat chakra affirmation:
I live an authentic life. I speak my truth.

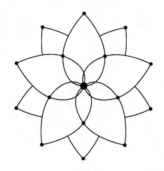

PART 8

MOVING YOUR THIRD EYE CHAKRA

*Dancing the third eye chakra has helped
me to trust my intuition more.
I feel like I've learnt a new language—one that has
more meaning than those I've known before.*

Corinne

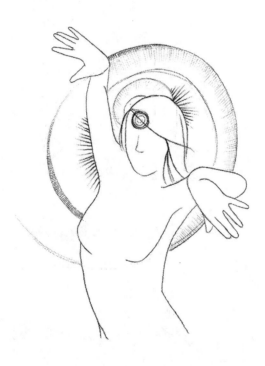

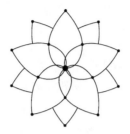

CHAPTER FORTY-EIGHT

the GIFT of INTUITION

The third eye chakra is the home of our intuition, also known as our sixth sense. Our intuition is like our own early-warning system, showing us where we are off track or off purpose, guiding us to where we need to be and showing us what we need to do. Even though this heightened sense is innate in all of us, many struggle to recognise it. And even when we do, we often fail to trust it.

Have you ever had the experience of just knowing you shouldn't do something, but then you went ahead and did it anyway? It may be something as simple as driving to work via a particular route. Your intuition tells you not to, then when you get stuck in a traffic jam for the next thirty minutes, you find yourself saying, 'I knew it! Why didn't I trust it?' Our intuition is always guiding us—from simple scenarios like this one to the critical decisions and important aspects of our lives.

Our intuition is a higher sense of perception. It gives us the ability to know something, even when we have no rational explanation for knowing it. It's like a source of wisdom that we receive in a flash. It can almost feel like seeing a shooting star. The flicker is so awesome, but then it quickly disappears. We can be left questioning whether we made it up. As there is no logical reasoning associated with it, we often tend to ignore it. The more we ignore these flashes, the less we notice them. We become disconnected from the powerful gift of our intuition.

As we balance our third eye chakra, we begin to notice these fleeting sensations more often and trust their messages. Following the breadcrumb trail of intuitive flashes can help guide our lives in powerful ways.

As I was writing this chapter, a public relations website I used to be a member of flashed into my mind. I had unsubscribed a couple years earlier and hadn't thought about it since. Following this flash, I immediately subscribed again. Ten minutes later, I received an email inviting me to apply for an amazing PR opportunity for Chakradance. By the end of the day, I had signed a contract and the events were in motion. Had I ignored that flash, none of this would have happened.

When we trust our intuition and act on it, everything just seems to flow. All the pieces come together effortlessly. We don't need to force things or try too hard. It's as if we're moving in rhythm with a higher power.

Albert Einstein once said: *The intuitive mind is a sacred gift and the rational mind is a faithful servant. We have created a society that honours the servant and has forgotten the gift.*

As we balance our third eye chakra, it's like we turn a light switch on in our lives, allowing us to see in new ways. We learn to balance our logical mind with our intuitive mind, so our lives become guided by both.

Developing our intuition also heightens our connection to what Carl Jung termed 'synchronicities.' Synchronicities are meaningful coincidences, like when we bump into an old friend who just happens to have a message we need to hear. Or we go into a bookshop, and the book we need to read falls off the shelf in front of us. When we find ourselves in the right place at the right time, we are in synchronicity.

As I was writing the above sentence, an old friend of mine texted me and happened to mention that he was re-reading his favourite book, *Synchronicity*. I couldn't help but laugh at the synchronicity of that!

Synchronicities are a bit like being tuned into a giant cosmic web. It's as if our souls attract the exact people, events and circumstances we need, to guide us on our path. What I have found interesting is that the more conscious we become of synchronicities, the more they seem to unfold in our lives. It's like a ripple effect. However, if we shut down this awareness, we often miss the opportunities being shown to us.

Balancing our third eye chakra increases our connection with coincidences and helps us to see the greater significance they play in our lives.

Meditation: *Awakening Your Intuition*

We all have intuitive abilities. I like to imagine our intuition as a muscle. The more we use it and develop it, the more powerful it becomes.

This is a very simple meditation that can help us strengthen our intuition and open us up to synchronicities in our lives. Before beginning this meditation, reflect on any situation in your life that you would like to gain more insight or clarity into.

You can do this meditation by reading the following steps, pausing after each one to imagine what has been described, or by listening to it with my voice-over guidance on the Third Eye Meditation: Awakening Your Intuition track: [refer to page vi]

1. Prepare your sacred space and yourself and then sit comfortably in quiet meditation. Gently close your eyes and focus on your breathing. Breathe a little more deeply and slowly than you usually do. Spend a few minutes focusing on your breath and letting everything slow down.

2. Imagine yourself sitting at the top of a mountain. It is nighttime and the sky is lit up with bright shining stars. You look up and find the brightest star, and you feel the light of that star shining down into your third eye chakra. It feels like an activation; an awakening of your intuition.

3. As your third eye awakens, you feel yourself gently floating up to your star. It feels peaceful and magical.

4. Bring into your mind a situation that you would like more insight or clarity on. See the details in your mind's eye. Observe the situation as though you were simply a witness looking on. From your position among the stars, you can see it all from a much higher perspective. Notice how clear your mind feels.

5. When you are ready, imagine surrounding the whole situation in a ring of starlight. Ask your higher self, your soul self, for a direct, intuitive experience about it in the near future. Now visualise the situation, still circled in starlight, leaving your mind. Let it go.

6. It's now time to gently float back down to the mountain top. Feel yourself sitting on the mountain. When you're ready, gently open your eyes and bring your awareness back into your space.

This meditation can be done as many times as you like. Each time you may choose to bring in a different situation that you would like intuitive guidance on.

Following the meditation, be open to receiving an intuitive experience or knowing, while also remaining slightly detached. Intuition is not something we can reach or grasp for. That would be like trying to catch light with our hands. It is more about creating space, about opening our hands to allow the light to come in. We need to be ready and open to receive.

I often find that I receive flashes of insight when I am doing something monotonous, like peeling vegetables, cleaning the house, or taking a shower. This slightly detached state opens me up to guidance. My children have even joked about getting me a whiteboard to go in the bathroom, as I often come running out to write something down after my shower.

After this meditation, you may receive a flash of insight while doing something monotonous. You might experience a chance encounter or hear a meaningful song. The people talking at the next table in a cafe may be saying exactly what you need to hear. An email may arrive.

I truly believe that if we ask for guidance we receive it. It may not always arrive in the way we are expecting. In fact, it rarely does. But it does come. Intuition is like electricity. We can't see it, but it does exist. Be open to experiencing it.

Once we receive an insight, it is powerful to anchor it in our physical realm. Write it down, paint it, sing it, move it, or whatever feels right to you. The aim is to bring our intuition into our daily life as much as we possibly can.

I've had some pretty remarkable experiences this week with the third eye chakra—lots of synchronicities and visions. My intuition is on.

Jill

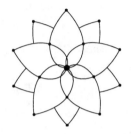

CHAPTER FORTY-NINE

the POWER of VISION

Just as balancing the throat chakra opens us up to clairaudience, the ability to hear clearly, so does the third eye chakra open us up to clairvoyance, the ability to see clearly. Many psychics see visions of the past and future, which gives them insight and guidance into situations in their lives and the lives of those around them. Dancing the third eye chakra helps us be open to these visions.

When Zabeth danced the third eye chakra, she saw some very frightening visions. She saw the world as complete pandemonium—earthquakes, the splitting of the earth, and death. She saw separation and loss, the failure of her marriage. Through her mandala, she also saw that there was hope.

Although frightening, in retrospect Zabeth felt that those visions were symbolically warning her, helping her to prepare for what was coming in her life—her mother and father-in-law's health crisis and the effect this had on her marriage. Her in-laws live on the other side of the world and Zabeth's husband had to travel across the world to help his parents, once a month on average, sometimes even more often. On one occasion, just as he landed back home, he received a text message that his mother had fallen and he had to turn and catch the next flight back. All this put enormous pressure on Zabeth's relationship with her husband. Her vision had shown her how this pressure might cause the death of their marriage.

The insight from her vision helped Zabeth to consciously choose a different way forward. She decided to support her husband and not ask him to choose between his parents and his marriage. She knows the risk that her marriage will fall apart continues to be there, but it's easier knowing that she is consciously working with the situation, not just letting her feelings overwhelm her and her behaviour. It's as if she can see the situation from a higher perspective and is acting from there.

These days, when her husband comes home completely burnt out, she is able to support him and express what a loving son he is being to his parents. She accepts that he needs to rest and restore when he comes home. Although Zabeth has fears of abandonment, her visions have helped her understand that her husband is not abandoning her. Instead, the way her husband treats his parents shows her that he is a faithful and dedicated person.

Our visions are there to help us, to show us the way towards resolution and growth. They often work symbolically. For example, seeing death may symbolise the death of a situation, rather than the death of a person. Likewise, birth can signify the birth of a project or an idea, rather than a baby. Seeing frightening images may symbolise the fear within us. The more we develop our third eye, the more meaning we will find in our visions.

Some of our visions even give us a direct look into the future. After Gail danced the third eye chakra, she drew a detailed mandala featuring a door. Some months later, when she was packing up her house to move, Gail's husband came across the mandala and asked her if she knew what it was. She told him that it was the door to her third eye. Her husband laughed and said, 'Don't you see what this is?' Gail went back into her memory of her dance but couldn't see what he, and also her children, were now seeing. Then she realised that the unusual door she had drawn was an almost perfect image of the door to the house they were moving into. She checked the date when she had drawn the mandala, and it was exactly one year to the day when contracts were finalised on their new home. Clearly, she had been intuitively guided towards her new home.

Visual imagery

Among the visions and images we see in our third eye are those we create through our imaginations. Here is a wonderful quote by the writer, Richard Bach: *To bring anything into your life, imagine that it's already there.*

The power of our imagination is something that many of us do not use to best advantage. In fact, I feel the opposite is true. Many of us unconsciously use our imaginations to create exactly what we don't want in our lives.

We all daydream at times. Our minds wander off, playing out different scenarios. Often a whole movie has unfolded on the inner screen of our third eye, before we catch ourselves and snap back into reality. We have unconscious loops that surface in our minds as we are driving or getting dinner ready. Sadly, a lot of our internal movies have negative images. They focus on a lack of something in our lives. Or we see problems, limitations and disasters. Many of us aren't aware that the images in our minds create scenarios in our real lives. We unconsciously use our imagination to give energy and power to our negative patterns, thereby drawing that kind of experience towards us.

The true power of our imagination is something that cannot be underestimated. The images we create in our minds set our future lives in motion. If we are constantly seeing problems, we will keep experiencing problems. To create the lives we want, we need to consciously shift the images in our minds.

Successful athletes constantly harness the power of their imaginations. When I was younger, I was a gymnast. I used to tour with a display team and we would do somersaults through fire rings and other risky tricks. Before I would raise my arms and take off to do a leap, I would always envision myself doing the trick. Somehow I knew that if I did it in my mind first, I would then do it for real.

I have heard this same story from many athletes, as well as people in other professions. Many business people (likely the most successful ones) imagine the meeting they are about to go into unfolding in exactly the right way. And then it does. Some lawyers do this, before getting up in front of a jury to make an argument. Public speakers have been known to do it before addressing a crowd. It's like envisioning the world as we would like it to be.

We use our third eye to create the blueprint for our future. Just imagine what happens when we keep giving our negative images more and more energy. As part of our self-healing, we need to learn how to use our imagination to create positive blueprints, so that we can manifest the lives we want.

Time to try: *Creative Visualisation*

It is now time to create a new blueprint—a positive image of how you would like your life to be. Before you begin your visualisation, reflect on what you would like to bring into your life. It's a good idea to start simply, then progress to deeper issues as you become more practised in the art of creative visualisation.

To begin with, you may want to improve a circumstance in your life or to have a positive outcome with some project you are working on:

1. It is best to do this exercise with your eyes closed. To begin, count down from ten to one, feeling yourself becoming more deeply relaxed with each count.

2. Imagine there is a movie screen in your mind's eye. The screen lights up, ready for the movie to begin. You see your name on the screen. Now picture the situation you thought of earlier playing out exactly as you would like it to. Feel free to rewind and change the movie, if it starts to go off in the wrong direction. You are the creator of this movie and in complete control. Spend as much time as you like, creating exactly what you want.

3. The key to successful creative visualisation is to imbue your images with feeling. Believe what you are seeing is happening and feel a sense of joy, love or whatever feeling is connected to your desired outcome.

4. When you feel you have created exactly what you need, complete the process with an intention. You may see this written up on the screen, like the credits of a movie. Or you may like to say the following intention silently or out loud to yourself: *This or something better now manifests for me in totally satisfying and harmonious ways, for the highest good of all concerned.* (This powerful intention is by Shakti Gawain, author of the book *Creative Visualization.*)

5. Let the screen slowly fade away. When you are ready, open your eyes and bring your awareness back into your space.

6. Following your creative visualisation, it helps to ground the imagery into your physical world. You may choose to do some journalling or find an object in nature that symbolises the new vision.

As you step back out into your life after this exercise, imagine the new scene as real and already accomplished. You're not just pretending; it's as though your new vision is happening now, in the present. You have created the blueprint and now the physical manifestation will follow.

As with anything in life, the more practice, dedication and integrity we apply, the more powerful the effect. Tune into your internal movie at least daily, and more often if you can. Creating a new blueprint takes time but is well worth the effort.

Time to try: *Vision Boards*

If you have difficulty visualising in your mind's eye, you can create a vision board. A vision board works in a similar way to visualisation in that it creates a new blueprint for us to step into. The only difference is that you create this blueprint in the outer world, instead of in your mind.

To create a vision board, you will need a pile of magazines from which you can take images and a board of some kind to stick the images on.

Before beginning, create your sacred space and set an intention of creating a vision for the highest good. Just as with creative visualisation, you may choose to focus on one aspect of your life—finances, relationships, health, spirituality—or you may choose to dedicate different sections of the board to different areas. Trust in what feels intuitively right for you.

While in your sacred space, spend some time flicking through the magazines and tear out any images or quotes that feel right for you. Be guided by your intuition. Your images may literally represent what you want to create in your life, or they may be symbolic and reflect the mood or energy of your vision. Sometimes you may not know why you have selected a particular image. If it feels right, just go with it. It may make more sense to you later on.

Once you have a collection of images that represent your ideal vision, stick them onto your board in a way that feels intuitively right for you. Display your vision board in a space where you will see it often. Then whenever you see it, you will end up doing short visualisation exercises throughout your day.

As with creative visualisation, imagine that what is on your vision board has already happened. Remember, this is your new blueprint and now the manifestation can take place.

As I danced the third eye chakra, there was a sense of past, present and future all being played out on my own personal screen, with a dream-like flickering of images.

Cinzia

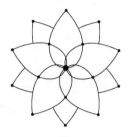

CHAPTER FIFTY

the MAGIC of YOUR DREAMS

The more we dance the third eye chakra, the more we begin to remember our dreams and value the messages they bring to us. When I began to study Jungian psychology, I discovered that one of the primary tools used is dream-work. I have to say that at first I was a little sceptical about putting so much trust and belief in the messages of our dreams. Having now done many years of dream-work, I am utterly convinced that this is one of the most fruitful ways of gaining deep insight into our lives.

Considering how much of our lives we spend dreaming, it's amazing that most of us attach little importance to understanding the symbolic messages delivered to us each night. I remember coming across this Jewish proverb: *An unexamined dream is like an unopened letter.* Making a commitment to spend a few minutes each morning reflecting on our dreams and inviting in the wisdom is a powerful way of working with the third eye chakra.

Our dreams are like messengers between our unconscious and consciousness. Imagine them as a bridge between our inner and outer worlds, as a thread linking our night and day. The messages are delivered in the form of symbols, images and metaphors, and each one has some wisdom and intuitive guidance to offer us.

I have to admit, it can be a slightly frustrating process when we first begin dream-work. We wake up grasping onto the flickering scenes of the night, and quite often they disappear into thin air so quickly. When we do manage to hold onto an image, our conscious mind immediately starts to try to make sense of it. But one of the most important things to keep in mind is that most dreams are probably not going to make literal sense. Dreams live in a realm unrestricted by time and space, so may be offering us insights about our past, present or future. Our dreams are symbolic and need to be approached from different angles. One of the quickest ways of blocking the insight is to try to make sense of these images with our logical mind because they are simply not logical.

Our dream life is made up of symbols that contain many layers of energy and different levels of meaning. There is an aliveness to a symbol, as it pulses with emotion, mood, memory and sensation. Symbols are the language of our unconscious. They give form to all this formless energy inside us.

When I was doing Jungian dream-work, the wonderful therapists I worked with would never try to analyse my dreams. They would ask me to close my eyes and guide me back into the dream imagery, so that I could reconnect with the feeling and mood. It's like being totally engrossed in a movie. We go back into the scene and feel the message. We feel the energy and the sensations in our body. This is our unconscious and consciousness dancing together. It doesn't mean that we will completely understand the dream, but there is a form of communication going on, one which was previously blocked.

Working with dreams

I encourage you to start doing your own dream-work. Keep a notebook and pen or pencil by your bed, so that you can record your dream experiences as soon as you wake. I've found it also helps to set an intention each night to remember our dreams.

Based on my studies and my own dream experiences, I have found that there are four different types of dreams, all of which we can work with in slightly different ways.

– ORDINARY DREAMS

The first kind just feels like an ordinary dream. They come to us like flashes of random episodes, as our unconscious sifts and sorts through the happenings of our previous day or prepares us for the day to come. We wake and have what feels like random pieces of a jigsaw puzzle flashing through our minds.

When you awake after an ordinary dream, record in your notebook as many facets of it as you can remember. It also helps to record what is going on in your daily life. I have found these ordinary dreams often give us guidance on what is happening for us right now. When we look at these dreams in the context of our daily life, we often gain insight into the messages. We won't always make sense of every aspect of the dream, but the more we nourish the communication between our inner and outer worlds, the more wisdom we gain.

To give a personal example, every so often I dream of wearing too much make-up. I don't normally wear a lot of make-up, so this dream never really made literal sense to me. When I started journalling about what had been happening in my life before having this dream, I started to notice that every time I had it, I had recently been acting in some way that was counter to my authentic self. I had been wearing a mask to try to fit in, or in some way pretending I was different to how I actually am.

Often we are unconscious of these kinds of behaviours. Now, whenever I have the make-up dream, I know that I am not being real in some part of my life and can consciously choose to step into authenticity.

– SIGNAL DREAMS

A few years ago, I had a dream that my brakes failed and I had a car accident. The next day, as I was driving past a service station, the dream flashed into my mind. I had my two young children in the car, so it was highly inconvenient to check it out. But the dream was vivid enough to make me take action. I explained to the mechanic that I had had a dream about my brakes failing, and I actually saw him roll his eyes. He checked everything out, then was quite apologetic as he told me that my brake fluid had run out. We could call this a coincidence, but when we are in the realm of intuition there is no such thing.

When working with signal dreams, it's important to remember that they can guide us on many levels, so we need to stay open to their messages. That's why, after having my brakes checked, I also reflected on where in my life I was failing to 'put the brakes on.' There were definitely areas where I really needed to slow down.

Even if you aren't sure whether you've had a signal dream, I recommend starting with the practical message. As Marion Woodman says: *If the dream says something is wrong with your body, check. Long before you do, your body knows when something is wrong.*

As with all dreams, record your signal dreams. We will often experience a number of signal dreams presenting the same message to us in various ways, until we finally receive it.

– BIG DREAMS

At other times, we have what I call 'big' dreams. These dreams have a completely different quality and intensity to them, and they stir something up inside us. They often have quite powerful symbolism and deep feelings or moods associated with them. Big dreams can also stay with us for days or months.

When we look at big dreams in the context of our daily life, they can seem to have no relation to our present circumstances. Instead, these big dreams can be about healing some aspect of our childhood or a past trauma in our lives. They can be about a wounded aspect of our feminine self or a denied part of our masculine self. When big dreams surface, our psyche is ready to begin the healing process.

Working with these dreams is a way of connecting with emotions and feelings that we have buried, slowly bringing them to the surface. As you wake after a big dream, spend some time staying with the dream imagery. Allow the feelings of the dream to stay with you. Sometimes when we have a big dream, we can't remember it, but we wake with the feeling, the intensity of the dream. This is the most important aspect. In your notebook, record those feelings as well as any images you remember. Write or use visual journalling, as a way of capturing the experience as best you can. Remember the bridge. The dream and the feelings it stirred up are a connection to your deep inner world.

Our big dreams will have lots of personal symbolism for us. We may dream of houses or people or our pets. Each symbol represents an aspect of ourselves. The house is our psyche. The people are different aspects of our personalities. Our pets are often our instincts or some other aspect of us. This can be challenging, as we will often feel like the dream is about the person we dreamt about, but our psyche is using that person as a symbol to show us a buried part of ourselves. Let your big dreams sink in. Let them stew. Give them time. You will have an aha moment, when you energetically receive the message of the dream.

— ARCHETYPAL DREAMS

More rare are the archetypal dreams that may come when we are at a deep crisis point in our lives, or when we are deeply engaged with our internal transformation. The symbols of these dreams are highly charged with energy and are not from our daily lives. Instead of day-to-day things like cars, houses or familiar people, these dreams include symbols like powerful snakes, strange animals or aliens. They may also include sacred geometry or religious symbolism.

A dream like this often serves as an initiation into a new aspect of our lives, and it tends to stay with us for many years. Part of why its energy is so big is because we are experiencing a process that is not just about us personally, but about being human. Many people before us have gone through this process of inner transformation, and it's as though our dream is energetically connecting us to the collective experience.

With this type of dream, it may be helpful to investigate dream symbols and their meanings. Often these dreams mirror messages from fairytales or myths, which can give an insight into the transformational process you are undertaking.

If you have an archetypal dream, treat it with respect. Like any other dream, record the experience and feel the emotions. Also, remember to trust that great inner transformation is at play in your life at that time.

Following any dream-work, I would recommend finding some way of anchoring the experience in your physical life. I often dance my dreams during the dance of the third eye chakra, by letting the images from them move through my body. Any form of creative expression can help give physical form to our unconscious.

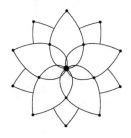

CHAPTER FIFTY-ONE

TRANCE DANCE

Dancing the third eye chakra has roots in the ancient practice of trance dance. Repetitive body movements, hypnotic beats and darkness (eyes closed) all serve to stimulate dancers into a trance state. Trance dance has been a vital part of shamanic and Eastern dance cultures for thousands of years, and is practised to promote spiritual awakening and heightened visions.

Trance dance helps us to become much more open to intuitive insights. It helps us to shift from the rational, logical and deductive left brain to the more intuitive, imaginative and visionary aspects of the right brain. It's like a doorway leading us into a non-linear world of mystery. In this heightened state, we open up to our internal guidance, as well as guidance from higher realms. We enter a state of timelessness, experiencing the past, present and future in the dance. We may even become open to connections with non-physical beings—relatives who have passed over, guides and angels.

When I was in my early twenties and backpacking around Europe, I discovered the world of nightclubs. Some of the experiences I had in these clubs were profound. As I danced with hundreds of people to repetitive beats, the feeling was hypnotic. The experience felt like trance dancing. Looking back, I think that many of the DJs were like urban shamans, guiding us into altered states of consciousness. The downside, of course, was that there was no safety. Back then, I can remember imagining what it would be like to dance that way in a safe and sacred space. I feel this is what the dance of the third eye is—a modern-day trance dance done in a sacred space.

When Rhiannon danced the third eye chakra, she felt as though she had fallen into a trance-like state. She found herself back in medieval days, wearing an indigo cape and riding alone on a white horse along a never-ending cobblestone path. On both sides of the path was a projection screen, playing scenes from her past and present. She could also see future scenes with maps for her to follow. The guidance she received from this dance gave her a clear sense of the direction she needed to take.

When Fiona danced the third eye chakra, she was going through a tough time with her partner. As the music started, pictures began to flood into her mind. She was running through rainforests, dancing around fire, just bang, bang, bang—one image after the other. Then she saw her boyfriend and herself. He was standing in their kitchen, and she ran towards him, jumping into his arms. Two large, beautiful wings unfolded from him as he took her in his arms, and they flew up into the sky. They flew through clouds and over mountain peaks. He held her tightly, and she felt so protected and safe. They landed on a mountain top surrounded by clouds, and then her wings unfolded. Their wings wrapped around each other, and she felt such love and peace.

Afterwards, Fiona went home and told her boyfriend about her vision, and they both smiled. Her vision confirmed the love and commitment in their relationship for both of them.

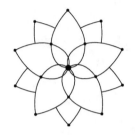

CHAPTER FIFTY-TWO

DANCING the THIRD
EYE CHAKRA

*As I danced the third eye chakra, I kept finding a
movement that worked well for a bit, then I needed
to change to another movement. Most of them
involved swinging or sweeping my arms in various
directions. As I was dancing I saw, and felt, a flash
of white light and felt like I'd crossed a barrier. I felt
a release. I felt more open and lighter. Then I felt
like I was moving through time and space, being
reminded of all the possibilities and no limits. I saw
how there is no need to rush; it's all in divine order.*

Sherri

It is now time to move your third eye chakra. There is a wonderful quote by Rumi: *Close both eyes ... look from the other
eye.* In many ways, that is what we will be doing in this dance.

Prepare your sacred space and yourself. Once you are ready, take three slow, deep breaths. Before you play the music, ask your higher self or higher guidance for what you need to see most right now. What insight, visions and/or guidance would be most helpful for you?

Now play the Move Your Third Eye Chakra music [refer to page vi]. Close your eyes and as you surrender into the beats, find your own movements. As images begin to unfold on your inner screen, you may find yourself expressing these images through movement.

What I've discovered in dancing the third eye chakra for many years is that we can't force anything to happen. The dance requires surrender, letting go. This can be challenging for many of us, because we are so used to controlling how we do things. Where we do have control is in preparing ourselves beforehand and setting a clear intention. We can then let go and become like an empty vessel, waiting to be filled. Through our dance, we become like a sacred cup waiting to receive the insight and the grace of wisdom.

The experiences that take place will be different for each of us and can be different each time we dance. Some of us will see images in our mind's eye or receive clear guidance, but not everyone experiences vivid visions when dancing the third eye chakra. We may instead have fleeting insights that contain the essence of other realms, or we may see flashes of light. We may experience waves of energy or physical sensations.

We may not consciously understand what is happening in the dance, and that's completely normal. We just need to trust that energy is moving through us. Often it is through the mandala, or events that take place after the dance, that we receive the insights we need.

The image for my mandala of the third eye chakra was of me holding my head back to the Universe. My shoulders are relaxed, my arms hanging down and back. My chest is open, my throat is open, my mouth is gently open. My hair is falling back and also being charged with indigo light—like an antenna. My eyes are closed, forehead to the sky and my third eye is open. The title that came to me was 'Eye Open' which I then realised was also 'I Open.'

Lisa Marie

Chanting the third eye chakra

The mantra sound for the third eye chakra is OM, which is pronounced as AUM. You might like to take a few minutes to try chanting this sound.

Sit peacefully and bring your awareness to your breathing. Inhale fully through your nose. As you exhale, vocalise the mantra OM, while focusing your awareness between your eyebrows.

Take notice of any feelings, memories, images or sensations that come up for you as you chant. Spend a few minutes coming back to your natural breathing to finish.

You can return to Chapter 44—Sacred Singing and Chanting, to revisit information on chanting the chakras.

Third eye chakra affirmation:
I trust my intuition. I see clearly.

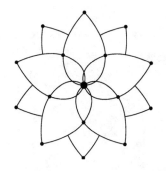

PART 9

MOVING YOUR
CROWN CHAKRA

The crown Chakradance was just beautiful. There was such a flow of energy coming from my crown, my heart and my hands. It brought tears of happiness as I danced. The message was: 'You are home.'

Leslie

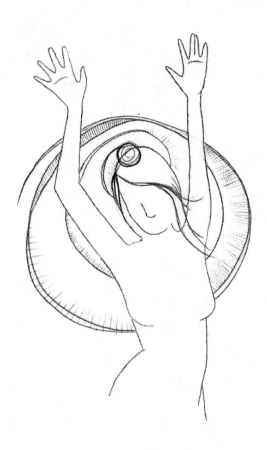

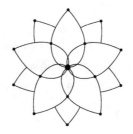

CHAPTER FIFTY-THREE

SOUL WISDOM

Our journey began by reconnecting with the wisdom of our bodies at the base chakra. Now, as we move into the crown chakra, we will find ourselves experiencing the wisdom of our souls.

The words of Deepak Chopra have always been very helpful to me in understanding the relationship between body and soul: *Essentially we are spiritual beings, made manifest in physical form. We are not human beings that have occasional spiritual experiences; rather, we are spiritual beings that have occasional human experiences.*

Balancing the crown chakra helps us to reconnect with our spiritual self, our soul, which is the essence of who we are. It's from here that we ask ourselves the question: *Who am I? Beyond my body, my job, my relationships, my home, my goals, who am I?*

I've always been fascinated by the idea of souls. Growing up in the Catholic Church, I learnt from our parish priest that every time we went to church we let a soul out of purgatory. This concept no longer resonates with me; but as a young child, the idea of souls being trapped in purgatory filled me with horror. After hearing this, I spent weeks using my lunch break at school to leap in and out of the church door, keeping count of the number of souls I thought I was releasing! I even recruited friends to help me with my mission.

When I was in my late twenties, I had a particularly powerful experience during a ten-day silent Buddhist retreat. It was day seven of meditation, when I suddenly found myself outside my body. I was up high, near the ceiling, looking down on my body and the rest of the people in the room. There seemed to be nothing strange about this at the time. I wasn't scared. On the contrary, I felt so light and free. I then wondered whether I could travel into the adjoining room and before I knew it, I was there. I quickly returned to the main meditation room because I didn't want to go too far away from my body. But I knew that if I had wanted to, I could have travelled anywhere. Next thing I knew, I was back in my body meditating again. Something changed in me forever that day. I had experienced my soul.

We've all heard stories about people who have had near-death experiences. They describe a similar kind of recognition of the eternal part of themselves. It's like we are wearing a particular set of clothes necessary for this life, but when the time is right, we respectfully release the garment of our body and move onto whatever comes next. Most people who have had a near-death experience tend to shift their perspective on how they want to live their lives. They bring their soul essence into everything they do. They often live their lives more fully. More soul-fully.

When I first danced the crown chakra, I had another powerful experience of connecting with my soul. This time I didn't leave my body. Instead I had an experience of my soul moving through my body. It felt as though a warm nectar was entering through the crown of my head and permeating my whole body. It felt like this nectar was moving my body. I heard the words 'Hello Natalie' and experienced a powerful recognition of the deeper part of me. In this dance, it felt like all my daily concerns just melted away. The stresses of my life felt insignificant. All the layers of what I thought defined who I was somehow dissipated. I moved beyond these and danced with the full presence of my soul.

Paradoxically, I found that letting go of the attachments to my physical world only improved it. When we let our soul move through us and guide us, we live our lives in a more sacred way. It's not about letting go of our responsibilities or caring less about our physical lives, it's that we seem to find more meaning and depth in our daily experiences. It's as though we approach our lives from a different place.

Many of us have lost connection with our soul. It's not something we often talk about or even consciously understand or recognise. We may just feel disconnected. Or there may be a vague sense of emptiness or meaninglessness in our lives. We may have become overly connected to our physical existence and lost connection with our spiritual essence.

In traditional shamanic cultures, it is believed that symptoms like depression, anxiety, addiction, compulsive behaviours and so on arise from a loss of connection with the soul. In our modern-day lives, these conditions are rife. Many of us either suffer in silence or take medication to numb the pain.

Many years ago, I heard a profound quote by thirteenth-century Persian poet, Rumi: *The wound is the place where the light enters you.* This gives us another way of looking at our symptoms. They are often the cries of our soul calling us to reconnect back to the deeper part of ourselves. They can be signs that we are trying to escape our soul's journey, rather than fully living it. Alcoholism, for example, was once described to me from a spiritual perspective as 'the search for Spirit in a bottle.' When we face our addictions, our restlessness, our anxieties and our wounds, we find the way back to our soul.

Judy had spent much of her life struggling with perfectionism and an addiction to working. She kept herself so busy and was so controlling of her life that she felt totally disconnected from any sense of her soul. When she danced the crown chakra, she found herself trying to perform, to dance well. But every time she tried to dance better, she felt a stronger force pushing her down to the ground. She finally got the message and stayed on the floor. She heard a voice say, 'Just be still.' In that moment, she felt the connection between her dance and her life. She could see how she was always trying to perform and make things perfect. She could see how she never took the time to be still and open to messages from the one source that always knew what was right for her—her soul.

Since dancing the crown chakra, Judy is more willing to slow down and trust the guidance she receives. She has been able to follow her purpose with less struggle. And while she feels much more connected to the soulful part of herself, she also feels much more comfortable in her own skin, in her body, and with who she really is.

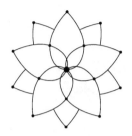

CHAPTER FIFTY-FOUR

BRINGING SACREDNESS INTO YOUR LIFE

A simple way of reconnecting with our soul is to invite sacredness into our daily life. There is a saying by Lakota medicine man, Black Elk: *As you walk upon the sacred earth, treat each step as a prayer.*

Sacredness will be different for each of us. Some of us may find it through religion and attend church or go to temple or mosque. For others, sacredness is found in the beauty and wonderment of nature. We may find it surfing a wave as we connect to the vastness of the ocean, or meditating in our own sacred space or on top of a mountain. We may find it by participating in ritual or ceremony.

It doesn't really matter how or where we find sacredness in our lives. What matters is that we connect with it and let it infuse our lives. We don't need to travel to ashrams or undertake spiritual initiations, unless we are deeply called to such things. It is enough to live the lives we have chosen with soulful awareness.

I have found a simple way to bring sacredness into our lives is to simply slow down, to do as Black Elk suggested and consider each step we take, making it our prayer. It sounds easy and it is, yet so many of us seem to struggle with it. Many of us charge through the day with little or no awareness of the beauty around us. When was the last time you stopped to smell a flower? Or lay on your back in the grass and watched clouds move into shapes? In many ways, sacredness is about simply being present. It's about appreciating the fullness of each moment in life, of each step we take.

Another simple but highly powerful way to bring sacredness into our lives is through gratitude. Give thanks as you eat your meals. Give thanks when your friends help you. Find gratitude for the small things each day. Even when we are struggling, we can always find at least one thing to be grateful for. It could be something as simple as the sun shining or the birds singing.

The mystic Meister Eckhart said: *If the only prayer you ever say in your entire life is thank you, it will be enough.* When we open to gratitude, we are closer to soul.

I remember coming across a book called *365 Gratefuls* that contained a collection of gratitude photos. It was by a woman named Hailey Bartholomew, and she took a photo of things she was grateful for, every day for one year. She suffered from depression and anxiety when she began the project. but by looking daily through the eyes of gratitude, her depression lifted and her appreciation of the world around her grew.

Gratitude connects us to the sacred, and the sacred connects us to soul.

Time to try: *Soul Time*

A powerful way to invite sacredness into our lives is to begin each day with a short ritual. Set aside five or ten minutes to intentionally honour your soul. You might light a candle or create your own altar, then spend some time in quiet meditation. Your ritual could include choosing a card from an oracle deck or reading a page or two from an inspirational book. You might simply spend a few moments setting an intention for the day. Whatever you choose, think of this time as soul time.

Following your morning ritual, spend a couple of minutes visualising your day ahead and ask your soul to guide you throughout it. You may want to include a talisman as part of your ritual. This could be a small crystal or a piece of jewellery that you hold onto during your morning ritual, then carry in your pocket or wear as you go about your day.

I often carry a talisman. I find that each time it catches my attention, I stop for a minute or so, breathe, and become more fully present in the moment. It helps me to tune back into my intention for the day and come back into alignment with my highest path. I encourage you to find or create your own talisman, as a way of bringing soul sacredness into your everyday life.

The more consistent I am with my soul time, the more my life flows. This daily time moves beyond being a nice thing to do and becomes an essential thing to do. Soul time puts our lives back into perspective. It opens us to our own internal guidance.

I am reminded of one of my favourite quotes by Swami Vivekananda: *You have to grow from the inside out. None can teach you, none can make you spiritual. There is no other teacher but your own soul.*

Meditation: *Soul Message*

During soul time, you might try this guided meditation. It helps connect us to our own inner healing sanctuary, a sacred space where we can connect with our soul.

You can do this meditation by reading the following steps, pausing after each one to imagine what has been described, or by listening to it with my voice-over guidance on the Crown Meditation Soul Message track: [refer to page vi]

1. Prepare your sacred space and yourself. Sit or lie down comfortably and spend a few minutes focusing on your deep breathing. Have the intention of releasing any tightness or tension in your body. Let any thoughts or worries drift away in a bubble of light.

2. Imagine that you are standing in front of a huge, ancient door. It is the most beautiful door you have ever seen in your life. It feels like this doorway has been there for many thousands of years, and you sense that you have passed through it many times. As you are wondering how you are going to open such a large door, it opens magically for you.

3. As you step through the door, you find yourself entering a beautiful, colourful garden. You can smell the most divine perfume. As you walk into the garden, you see a waterfall cascading into a gentle river. The water is sparkling, as though tiny crystals are dancing in it. You feel drawn to take off your clothes and stand under the waterfall. You feel the tiny crystals gently massaging away any heaviness or tiredness. Anything that you are carrying can now be released. Spend as long as you need under the crystal waterfall.

4. As you step out, you find a white robe waiting for you and you wrap it around yourself. You feel totally relaxed and safe. You notice a winding staircase on the other side of the garden. You can't see where it leads, as there is a golden mist

all around it. You walk over to the staircase and feel as though you are floating up the stairs. As you emerge at the top, you find yourself entering a magnificent temple. It is shimmering and sparkling, and appears to be made of crystals. You step inside and let the light infuse you. You can't remember ever feeling calmer or more relaxed.

5. In the centre of the temple is a large comfortable chair, and in front of it is a small table with an ornate book on it. You sit in the chair and see that the book has your name embossed on the cover. You pick up the book, knowing that there is a message inside for you. When you are ready, open the book and receive the message.

6. When the time feels right, place the book back on the table and imagine your eyes closing as you rest in the chair. You feel a presence above you and around you. It feels like a beautiful, golden angel. In this moment, you know that this presence is you. The golden light of your soul is like a warm nectar holding you. You now invite your soul to merge with you. Feel the light and radiance infusing you. Spend as much time as you need. Know that your soul is always with you.

7. When you are ready, give thanks and slowly step out of the temple. The golden mist clears as you slowly move back down the staircase. You pass back through the brightly-coloured garden, past the waterfall, towards the large door. Once again, the door opens for you and you step back out.

8. Take three deep breaths and slowly bring your awareness back to your sacred space.

This is a meditation that you can return to again and again. You may find other images begin to appear for you. You may receive different messages in the book. The language of your soul will deepen as your commitment to soul time deepens.

As with all inner work, it is most powerful when we do some kind of physical action afterwards, to bridge our inner experience with our outer world. Following this meditation, you may choose to write down the words you saw in the book. You may choose to paint the golden angel or your experience of it. You may choose to take a walk outside and find a feather or a stone, some object that symbolically represents the experience you've had. Simply have the intention of bringing your soul essence into your physical world and see what comes.

When I danced the crown chakra, I felt my
Mom and Gran holding my hands. It was so
moving, so light, and just what I needed.

Caithe

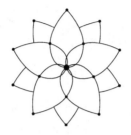

CHAPTER FIFTY-FIVE

SOUL CONNECTIONS

Dancing the crown chakra opens us up to experiences connected to this world and beyond. It's as though the veil between the worlds becomes thinner. Many people who have danced the crown chakra have shared their experiences of connecting with friends or relatives who have passed over. For some, there is simply a beautiful feeling or sense of the person being with them as they dance. For others, it can be a profound opportunity for some deep healing to take place.

Doreen's first husband died in a car accident as a result of his drinking. He was an alcoholic. Doreen, who was in her twenties at the time, always felt that she could fix him. She truly loved him and was constantly encouraging him to go to a rehab centre or seek some other kind of treatment. She was devastated when he died and felt like she had failed him in some way. She never got the closure she needed.

When Doreen danced the crown chakra, she saw her husband standing in front of her. He kept apologising for leaving her and for the way he had treated her. As she danced, she could see all the reasons why he felt the need to drink and why she was unable to help him. They cried, laughed and smiled together. He then drifted upwards in front of her and she felt as though she had complete closure at last.

Doreen continued to dance the crown chakra and each time experienced a release from soul encounters that had been holding her back. Towards the end of her dance a beautiful diamond appeared, which she took as a replacement for all the things she had let go. She felt a profound sense of freedom, happiness and joy.

I personally had a profound soul connection experience about eleven years ago, when I danced the crown chakra. It was one of my first experiences of being led by another facilitator in a live Chakradance class. As I danced, I felt the strong presence of a boy. I could feel his energy very clearly. When I asked who he was, he told me he was my son. It was a very moving experience. Exactly twelve months later, my son Tom was born. I knew instantly that this was the soul I had connected with in my dance.

As you dance the crown chakra, be open to the presence of your loved ones dancing with you. The experience can be truly blissful.

I danced the crown chakra today and I was reminded that I am constantly surrounded by divine energy, spirits, angels, love and light. I just need to open myself up to it.

Sheridan

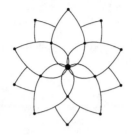

CHAPTER FIFTY-SIX

OPENING to SPIRIT

Whether we are religious or not, most of us believe in a power or source greater than ourselves. Some call it God, Buddha, Spirit, The Creator or the Divine Source, and there are countless other names. However we choose to label it, having a connection with a spiritual source is essential for a healthy life. In the words of Buddha: *Just as a candle cannot burn without fire, men cannot live without a spiritual life.*

Balancing the crown chakra involves making a commitment to our own spiritual practice. Our practice doesn't have to be elaborate or complicated. It can be simple and sacred. It doesn't need bells and whistles. It needs pure intention. The main thing our spiritual practice needs is consistency. Remembering that we are spiritual is a daily honouring. The late Wayne Dyer once said: *Heaven on Earth is a choice you must make, not a place you must find.* Committing to our spiritual practice is this choice.

One of the great blessings that comes from deepening our spiritual practice is the realisation that we don't need to rely on our own strength alone. We find that there is help and guidance available to us, if only we ask. A spiritual practice shows us that we don't need to push, control or force our way through life. We can surrender our challenges to a higher source and receive divine solutions.

This is both a comforting and empowering conclusion to come to, even though the outcomes may not always be as we envisioned. In fact, they rarely are. There is usually a divine plan far greater than anything we could have created or even imagined for ourselves.

Several years ago, my husband and I found ourselves having to sell our family home in Sydney. The moving date was fixed, the van was booked, yet we had no idea where we were going. Although I could sense that this was happening for a reason, I couldn't figure out why. As the date got closer, I became increasingly stressed and anxious. I was trying to figure out what to do and I was getting nowhere.

Just when I was near breaking point, I realised how much I was relying on my own strength to get me through. For some reason, I had abandoned my spiritual practice in my time of need. That day I returned to my practice and prayed for divine help. I surrendered my fear, anxiety and control over to Spirit and asked to be shown the way.

After that, I stopped running around trying to make things happen. Instead, I returned to my practice each morning. A few days later as I was meditating, I heard a sound at the front door. I had just asked to be shown guidance, so I immediately went to the door to see what had been delivered. I didn't really expect Spirit to deliver the answer direct to my doorstep, but I went to check anyhow.

I opened the door to find a brochure promoting a competition to win a family holiday in Noosa, a magical place in Queensland, Australia. When my husband and I lived in London many years ago, we used to spend a few days relaxing in Noosa every time we visited Australia, just because we found it so beautiful and peaceful. As I looked at that brochure, I had an aha moment of knowing. I could just feel that this was where we were now supposed to be. Within days, we had found a place to live and a school for our children, and we moved shortly after.

Five years later we are still in Noosa, and I have no doubt that this is our spiritual home. I feel deeply connected to the land and the people here, and my spirituality has deepened significantly. I hadn't been to Noosa in more than fifteen years before moving here, and I know I wouldn't have thought of it as a place to live if I hadn't been presented with that brochure. I feel I was guided by Spirit to the exact place I need to be.

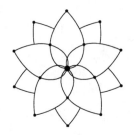

CHAPTER FIFTY-SEVEN

DEVELOPING YOUR
SPIRITUAL PRACTICE

There are many ways of developing a spiritual practice. Our practice can be whatever we want it to be, so long as it is regular and connects us to a power greater than our own. For some of us, our practice will be connected to our faith in a particular religion. For others, it may be connecting with spirit guides or angels. It may be through meditation or communing with nature. We may even find many different ways of connecting with a higher source throughout our lives. If you are searching, you might like to try the following spiritual practices.

Prayer

Prayer allows Spirit to offer us assistance in our lives. Prayer allows us to align our will with a higher will. In the words of Mother Teresa: *Prayer is not asking. Prayer is putting oneself in the hands of God, at His disposition, and listening to His voice in the depth of our hearts.*

When our lives feel challenging, overwhelming or confusing, simple prayers like *Thank you for showing me a way through this* or *Thank you for showing me a divine solution for this* are ways of surrendering to the higher guidance of Spirit.

A way of staying in alignment with our highest spiritual path can be to offer a prayer each morning, along the lines of: *Thank you for showing me how I can best serve the world today.*

In many ways, prayer is an act of surrender. Many of us struggle with surrender, because it can feel like an act of weakness. It can feel like we are letting go of control over our lives. For certain aspects of our lives we do need control, but for our spirituality, we need to learn the sacred act of surrender. We need to trust that Spirit is guiding us in the direction we need to go. Prayer can help us with this.

Prayer is something that we can also use to help others. We may pray for the safety for our children, our partners, our even someone we have never met.

A couple of years ago, I went to see the author Carolyn Myss at an event. She told a moving story about a woman who had been driving along a freeway, when she had an accident. She lifted out of her body and could see herself and the wreckage below her. The accident had caused a huge traffic jam, and she was witnessing all the chaos beneath her. She could hear lots of different voices speaking, most of them complaining about the hold-up, or raging that they were going to be late. Over the babble of complaints, she heard another voice praying. A woman way back in the traffic jam was praying that whoever was in the accident would be okay. As the woman who had left her body heard this, she went to see who this person was. She clearly saw the woman, sitting in her car and praying. The next minute she was back in her injured body and shattered car. She was taken to hospital and she survived.

After this experience, she could still clearly remember everything that had happened to her. She could even remember the licence plate on the car of the praying woman. Several weeks later when she got out of hospital, she contacted the woman and went to personally thank her for her prayers and for saving her life.

Since hearing this story, whenever I hear of an accident or of someone with an illness, I immediately offer my prayers.

Meditation

Meditation is a wonderful tool for helping us clear the chatter of our minds and open up to receiving divine guidance. There are different methods of meditation, two of which I've outlined below. Use whichever works best for you, do them both, or find a method of your own. Whatever practice you choose, the intention behind meditation is to become an empty vessel, waiting for the wisdom of Spirit to enter.

– SITTING MEDITATION

Sit comfortably and softly close your eyes. Breathe in and out through your nose, keeping your awareness with your breath, as it enters and leaves your nostrils. Any time you catch your mind wandering, simply let your thoughts go and bring your awareness back to your breath. You may sit in quiet meditation for ten or twenty minutes, or for however long feels comfortable for you.

As we deepen our practice of meditation, we begin to align ourselves with our soul self, our witness self. It's as though we can watch the crazy dramas going on in our minds, but become detached from them. The more we can detach and let them go, the more our mind begins to quieten. We begin to create the space to receive higher guidance.

— MOVING MEDITATION

If you find it difficult to sit in meditation, this moving meditation based on a Tantric energy exercise is a great alternative. It works best if you can give yourself enough time to really allow yourself to surrender to the experience. I recommend setting aside fifteen to twenty minutes if you can, but go with however much time you have available. The activity or action involved is in the preparation. We prepare our bodies and set an intention of opening to Sprit. We then actively let go and surrender. The surrender needed here is an active surrender; an undoing. In Buddhism it's called 'no mind' and in Taoism it's called 'action-less activity.' The more we achieve these states of deep surrender, the more we experience the Divine within ourselves.

Begin by creating your sacred space, internally and externally. Stand with your feet shoulder width apart. Feel your feet firmly on the ground beneath you. Have your knees slightly bent and your whole body loose. Softly close your eyes and take three deep breaths. Set the intention of being open to the grace and wisdom of Spirit, the Divine, God or whatever name you feel most comfortable with. Let go of any expectations.

Now, do nothing. Nothing at all. Keep coming back to your body and checking that it is totally loose and that you are not holding any tightness anywhere. Let it go and wait. Keep your feet firmly planted on the ground, but everything else loose. Feel as though you are waiting for an important visitor. Feel as though you are wakefully resting.

After a while, you will find that your body begins to make small movements on its own. Just observe these movements and go with them. You don't need to control them, change them, or understand them in any way. Just let these natural movements happen. After more time, you may find the movements get bigger or wilder. Or you may feel like making sounds. You may begin to sense a subtle energy connecting with you. You may feel tingling sensations or just feel slightly different from how you usually do. Enjoy the experience. When you are ready, take three deep breaths and come back into your space.

This form of meditation can take some practice. You may find on some occasions that you don't experience much other than a sense of calmness. On other occasions, you may have mystical experiences and receive divine guidance. We can't think or force our way to spiritual experiences, we can only create space ready to receive spiritual guidance. I believe this is what inspiration is. It is when we have silenced our internal chatter enough to be able to receive messages and wisdom from Spirit. When we are inspired, we are in Spirit.

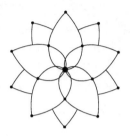

CHAPTER FIFTY-EIGHT

STAYING OPEN to
SPIRITUAL GUIDANCE

In addition to having a regular spiritual practice, we can set an intention for ourselves of being open to receiving and trusting spiritual guidance in our daily lives.

I heard a story many years ago that demonstrates how this can work ... or not. It is a story about a man who was a firm believer in God. The story goes something like this:

One day it began to rain heavily. The rain continued until there was a big flood coming. A neighbour knocked on the man's door and said, 'A flood is coming, you better get out with me while you can.' The man said, 'No, God will save me.' An hour later, as the floodwaters began to rise, a rescue worker paddled by in a boat. He said to the man, 'Get in this boat and ride to safety.' The man again replied, 'No, my faith is strong. I know God will save me.' The waters began to overtake the house and the man climbed onto the roof. A man in a helicopter hovered low, dropped down a line, and said, 'Grab hold of this rope and we will fly you to safety.' The man again replied, 'I'm fine, God will save me.' Then the man drowned. When he got to heaven, he said to God, 'I had such faith in you. Why didn't you save me?' God replied, 'I sent you a warning, a boat and a helicopter. What more did you want?'

As we begin to rely on a power greater than our own, we need to be open to the signs and messages we receive. Sometimes we expect that help and guidance will be shown to us in a specific way, or we expect it to be very obvious, but often guidance comes to us in small ways. Part of deepening our spiritual practice is heightening our awareness around the small signals we receive, then acting on them.

We are spiritual beings, but we are also human beings. Our life is a journey and we will each be thrown different obstacles and spiritual assignments along the way. Many of us will detour off the divine path. I know that I do quite frequently. And that's okay. That's part of being human. As we balance the crown chakra, we learn how to come back to the path more quickly and easily.

We may go for days or weeks when we are disconnected from our spiritual practice, then something jolts us back to remembering that we are spiritual beings having a human experience. It's when we wander off the path for years that we begin to experience the symptoms of our crying soul.

Maintaining a spiritual practice is such a powerful way of ensuring that we never wander too far and that our comeback rate is fast. A daily prayer you might like to try is: *I welcome the energy of Spirit to work through me today.* Or find your own daily prayer that helps keep you on track.

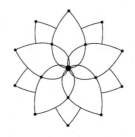

CHAPTER FIFTY-NINE

DANCING the CROWN CHAKRA

When I danced the crown chakra, I felt filled with peace. My overwhelming sense was of a blissful unity, a connection to all things. I felt a sense of joy for being who I am. During the dance, my feet were firmly rooted but my upper body swayed. My arms were weaving violet-coloured patterns of energy. I felt a ball of golden energy form in between my hands. It was made of Universal nectar. I let this build and then released it to the ether with healing intent. It floated upwards and continued to grow. I continued forming energetic 'balls' and towards the end of the dance I crouched down to the earth, releasing this healing energy downwards into the Mother. I had a strong sense of uniting the spiritual with the physical. The dance left me with the overriding sense that 'being' authentically myself automatically has a positive and healing effect on the Universe.

Gilly

It is now time to move your crown chakra. The dance of the crown chakra is a dancing prayer—an honouring of our soul as it moves through the sacred temple of our body. It is a divine moving meditation, connecting us with Spirit.

Create your sacred space and prepare yourself for this devotional dance. Once you are ready, take three slow, deep breaths and play the Move Your Crown Chakra [refer to page vi]. As you surrender to the music of the highest and most spiritual frequencies, you may experience the world beyond this one. You may find your consciousness expanding, reaching higher states of awareness. You may find yourself glimpsing the mysteries and the wonder of Spirit.

As you dance, you may feel a sparkling cord of light pulling ever so smoothly, ever so gently, from the top of your head— almost like an umbilical cord connected to the crown of your head. You may look up and see that this cord travels high up into the sky and is connected to the whole Universe.

Through the dance of the crown chakra, we physically embody Spirit. You may find your movements evoke the spiritual, such as finding the prayer position with your hands or raising your arms and hands up to receive Universal light. You may experience the light of your soul, like a nectar entering through your crown and permeating your whole body. The dance of the crown chakra is the soul's turn to dance.

Once you have finished your dance, take three slow, deep breaths, then sit down to create your mandala art.

*When I danced the crown chakra, Archangel Michael
appeared with a blue heart on the centre of his
majestic body. He was holding his sword. He handed
me the sword and instructed me to cut threads of
the past, which I did in a frenzied release. Towards
the end of the dance I felt hot, and words like
'surrender,' 'healing' and finally 'wholeness' embraced
my psyche. I named my mandala 'wholeness.'*

Moira

Chanting the crown chakra

The mantra sound for the crown chakra is NNGG (as in sing).
You might like to take a few minutes to try chanting this sound.

Sit peacefully and bring your awareness to your breathing.
Inhale fully through your nose. As you exhale, vocalise the mantra
NNGG, while focusing your awareness at the top of your head.

Take notice of any feelings, memories, images or sensations
that come up for you as you chant. Spend a few minutes coming
back to your natural breathing to finish.

You can return to Chapter 44: Sacred Singing and Chanting,
to revisit information on chanting the chakras.

Crown chakra affirmation:
*I am connected to and supported by
everything in the Universe.*

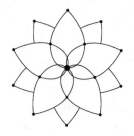

AFTERWORD

*I am living again. I love Chakradance. Life
has opened up and I feel so much lighter. My
appreciation for myself, and my life, is amazing.
I feel more like me than I ever have.*

Tracey

Congratulations on completing your journey through your
chakras. By now you will be feeling the changes in your life.
Some of them may be subtle and others may be profound. You
may be noticing shifts in your body, in your emotions and in
your relationships. You may be feeling more connected to your
passion, your purpose and your soul.

My hope is not only that your life has transformed in positive
ways, but also that you have stepped into a new way of living.
Chakradance and the tools and techniques in this book are not
just something you do once and tick off; they are practices you

can use for life. You will deeply benefit from them from the very start, but it is when you commit to practising them regularly that you will experience the most profound shifts in your life.

I encourage you to return to this journey again and again, as each time you dance, a little more blocked energy unravels and a little more energy flows. Dance by dance, you will feel like you are coming home to your true, authentic self.

I remember being very moved by how the great artist Michelangelo described creating his beautiful sculpture of David: *I saw the angel in the marble and carved until I set him free.* This feels to me like a beautiful metaphor for Chakradance—as we dance our way through our chakras, we keep peeling back the layers until we discover our own radiance, our own true nature within.

The practice of Chakradance

Our journey back to our authentic self is not linear, it's cyclical. We may experience some defining moments, but we need to choose consciousness again and again and again. Sometimes it feels easier to fall back to sleep and let the treadmill of life take over. But if we stay committed to our Chakradance practice, it becomes the guiding light on our journey, always leading us to where we need to go.

You can use Chakradance as your regular practice in many different ways. Some suggested ways follow, all of which I have personally used. I find that at different times in our lives we can use the practice in different ways. For example, when my children were very young, my practice was more limited than it is today, simply because I had less time to spare. The key is to be consistent about using the practice in some way. Listen to your own body, to your own soul, and be open to finding a rhythm that works for you.

– WEEKLY PRACTICE

A powerful way of practising Chakradance is to focus on **one chakra per week**. I find it's best to start at the base chakra and travel up to the crown, week by week. With a weekly practice, you may choose to dance the chakra you are experiencing every day, or just a couple of times a week. You may choose to revisit the meditations and exercises in the book again, and notice the shifts that are taking place. I would encourage you to continue journalling and reflecting on how your outer life connects to the chakra you are exploring. When our inner and outer lives are dancing together, we find flow in our lives.

Once you have journeyed through the chakras, you can return to the beginning and repeat the cycle. Each time you return, you will go a little deeper, discover a little more. Each dance will lead you closer to the core of who you are.

Another way of committing to a weekly practice is by **focusing specifically on a chakra that you know needs attention in your life**. Perhaps you are grappling with very low self-esteem, and something has come up in your life where confidence and personal power are really needed. In this situation, you may choose to focus on dancing the solar plexus chakra that week.

Although this is a powerful way to use Chakradance, I would recommend returning at some point to dancing all seven chakras on a regular basis, as a way of balancing your whole system.

– DAILY PRACTICE

You may choose to commit to Chakradance as a daily practice, and dance one of the seven chakras on each of the seven days of the week, being mindful of how your day unfolds in the energy of each chakra. If you have time, you may include the chakra meditations in your daily practice, as a way of deepening your experience.

As with the weekly practice, you may choose to focus on one particular chakra in preparation for something going on in your life. For example, you may want to dance the throat chakra, if you are doing some public speaking that day.

Another daily rhythm is to dance all seven chakras, from base to crown, one after the other in a single session. You can do this every day if you have time (it takes about an hour in total), or a few times a week. If you choose to do this, I recommend creating a mandala representing your whole system each time, and witness the transformations taking place.

– LIVE CHAKRADANCE CLASSES

If there is a Chakradance facilitator near you, I would encourage you to experience a live Chakradance class. Chakradance facilitators provide a sacred and nurturing space, and will **hold the space for you** as they guide you into your dance. Although live classes are still very focused on your personal journey, you will experience the power of group energy. When a group of people come together with the sacred intention of healing, the energy magnifies and deep transformational shifts often take place.

To find out if there is a class near you, go to Chakradance. com/find-a-Chakradance-class.

The dance of life

Our journey through this book has been focused on the journey within. Of course, this is only a part of our journey here in life. We are not islands. We have formed relationships with other people and are making our unique contribution to the world. All our experiences in the outer world will be affected by the inner journey we have taken (and will hopefully continue to take). Our experience of the outer world is at its best when we are coming from our authentic, whole self.

If we are disconnected and shut down within ourselves, it's very difficult to make a genuine connection with others or to find our true purpose in life. When we move our chakras and balance our energy, we are magnetically drawn towards people and opportunities that are in alignment with who we really are. This doesn't mean that we won't still face challenges in our lives, but we will be able to meet those challenges from a more authentic and real place.

We are all here on this planet together and we all impact on each other's lives. As we become more conscious and authentic, that energy ripples out to the people around us and calls them to do the same. There is a wonderful saying by Ram Dass that I love: *We're all just walking each other home.*

I would like to thank you from the bottom of my heart for joining me on this path. It has been an honour to guide you on this journey. Namaste.

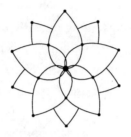

MAP of the CHAKRAS

CHAKRA	PHYSICAL LOCATION	BALANCED	IMBALANCED
Base	Base of spine/ perineum/ bones/ legs/ feet/ teeth/ large intestine/adrenals	Good overall physical health/ grounded/ stable/ feeling at home and safe in the world	Poor physical health/ out of touch with reality or overly materialistic/ overweight or noticeably underweight/ issues around money
Sacral	Lower abdomen/ ovaries or testes/ reproductive and urinary systems	Healthy sexuality/ able to feel and express emotions/ easily able to surrender to the flow of life/ finds pleasure in life	Sexual dysfunction/ over-emotional or lacking in feeling/ life feels flat or there is too much drama/ lack of passion or overindulging in life's pleasures
Solar Plexus	Middle abdomen/ digestive system/ pancreas/ muscles	Healthy digestion/ strong sense of inner strength and personal power/ reliable/ enjoys spontaneity and laughter	Poor digestion/ lack of energy/ undisciplined or obsessive about pursuits/ weak-willed and withdrawn or over-dominating and controlling
Heart	Centre of chest/ arms and hands/ heart/ respiratory system/ thymus gland	Compassionate/ able to form loving relationships/ able to feel self-love/ balanced outlook on life/ forgiveness comes easily	Lack of self-love/ jealous and possessive/ co-dependent or distant and unable to let people get close
Throat	Throat/ ears/ nose/ jaw/ thyroid and parathyroid/ neck/ vocal cords	Clear and truthful communication/ creatively expressive/ good at listening/ life feels harmonious	Unable to express true feelings/ fear of speaking or dominating conversations/ engages in gossip/ creatively shut down or blocked
Third Eye	Centre of forehead/ eyes/ pineal gland	Intuitive/ imaginative/ easily able to see the bigger picture/ good memory/ remembers dreams easily	Mental confusion/ limited view of life/ nightmares and hallucinations/ poor memory
Crown	Top of head/ brain/ central nervous system/ pituitary gland	Connection to spirituality/ a sense of sacredness in life/ regularly finds gratitude	Lack of meaning in life/ limited worldview/ sense of alienation/ spiritual addiction or little regard for anything of a spiritual nature

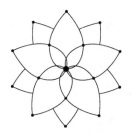

ACKNOWLEDGEMENTS

I would like to say a big thank you to the many wonderful people who have helped and supported me, not only in the creation of this book, but also in the development of Chakradance.

Special thanks to my husband, Paul, who believed so much in what I was doing that he left the world of advertising five years ago, to bring his marketing expertise to Chakradance. He is always there to support me and our global tribe of facilitators. Thanks also to our children, Lily and Tom, not only for their understanding during the many hours when I disappeared into my office to write, but also for being my constant teachers. Thanks to my mum, Mary, and my pop, Max, for all the babysitting and for nurturing me as I wrote this book. Thanks also to my dad, Kevin, for encouraging my love of music and to father-in-law, Robert, for all you have done to support me.

This book has been brought to musical life by the multi-talented Dale Nougher. Dale is a platinum-selling recording artist, pianist, composer and performer, and I am totally blessed that he has joined Chakradance full-time to work with me in composing our music. Thank you Dale, not only for the gift of your music, but also for your unwavering dedication and commitment to this journey we are on.

Thank you also to Ian Hildebrand, for many hours in the recording studio getting the voice-overs and the sound levels just right.

Great appreciation goes to my editor, Christa Bourg. Thank you Christa, for the care and attention you have given to every page of this book, as well as for being a constant guiding light for me throughout this writing journey. I have felt very held and supported by you the whole way through.

For over a decade now, I have had ongoing encouragement and support from Leon Nacson of Hay House Australia, who has made the publishing of this book possible. Thanks Leon, to you and your wonderful team.

A huge thanks to Stefanie Thompson for the beautiful illustrations throughout this book, to Tess Peni for the cover photography, and to Yanni Van Zijl for the magical photos you create for me.

In the pages of this book are real stories and experiences from some of the beautiful souls who practise, and in many cases now facilitate, Chakradance. I would like to thank each of you deeply, for sharing your vulnerability and pain as well as your transformations. I have no doubt that your stories will bring healing and hope to many.

To my friend, work partner and soul sister Anna Kelly, thank you for living the pages of this book with me and for being alongside me on this journey. I can't imagine doing it without you. Deep thanks also to my great friend and colleague, Jenny

Curtis, not only for supporting our tribe of facilitators, but for all you do for both me and Chakradance.

Chakradance would not be what it is today without the many years of blood, sweat and tears that Douglas Channing has poured into it. You are forever in my heart, Douglas. Gratitude also to Bronwyn Fish for your support and input in the early days of Chakradance. I'll always remember those days.

With a warm heart, I deeply thank every one of our Chakradance facilitators, for helping me share our practice with the world. The passion, dedication and commitment you all have inspires me every day. I can't imagine a more beautiful tribe to be part of. In particular, I would like to thank those who have also helped with training and translating: Sharon Hooper, Gail Johnson, Wendy Bradshaw, Susanne Danielson, Nicola Goddard, Veronique Thomman, Monique Mahn and Line Leduc, as well as Christina 'Tina' Davidson for all the wonderful blogs you have written for Chakradance.

Throughout my life, I have been fortunate to have many great teachers and guides. Thank you to everyone at the College of Psychic Studies who shared their wisdom with me, in particular Sue Allen and Linda Kay. Thank you to Beverly Martin, my teacher of Jungian Studies at the Society for Psychology and Healing. One of my proudest moments was when you shared with me that you thought Carl Jung would be well pleased with the development of Chakradance.

Enormous thanks to Carren Smith and my amazing mastermind buddies: Angela Counsel, Juliet Dyer, Michelle Mounsey, Marijana Marusic Jurgec, Sam Parker, Sabeeha Mailanji and Madhi Mason. Thanks to each of you for your ongoing support and guidance.

Two women who have played an enormous role in my life are my Jungian therapists, Sally Gillespie and Elizabeth Meakins. Words cannot express how grateful I am to you both.

I have been extraordinarily blessed to dance through life with a tribe of special friends dotted across the globe. Thank you Lea-anne and Dave Crawford, Krista Fergusson, Tracy French, Alana Fairchild, Rebecca Tapp, Lynette Sheldon, Lorella Ricci, Lisa Hewson Mollard, Kira Ivanoff, Amanda O'Dea, Kirsten Spry, Alison Bell, Justine Southgate and Karlie Francisco. Your friendship and support means the world to me.

I have found wisdom and inspiration in the pages of many books, but I especially want to acknowledge and thank Anodea Judith (*Wheels of Life*), Barbara-Ann Brennan (*Hands of Light*), Clarissa Pinkola-Estes (*Women Who Run with the Wolves*) and Marion Woodman (*Dancing in the Flames*).

I am deeply grateful for the encouragement and practical support I have enjoyed from Deepak Chopra, Tami Simon, Mark Metz, Jono Fisher, Lawrence Ellyard and Matt Howe.

Finally, I would like to thank each and every one of you who have joined me in the practice of Chakradance. I feel honoured to be on this journey with you.

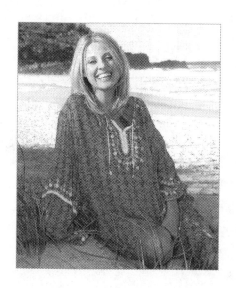

ABOUT the AUTHOR

Natalie Southgate created Chakradance (chakradance.com) in 1998, combining her training in dance, psychology and chakra healing to create this new fusion of modern music and ancient wisdoms. She has run Chakradance all over the world, including workshops at The Chopra Center in California and at Doreen Virtue's Angel Intuitive courses across Australia.

After many years of leading Chakradance, Natalie developed a training program so that others could facilitate this healing modality across the world. The tribe of Accredited Chakradance Facilitators now comprises over 500 beautiful souls in over forty countries, and is growing every year. For more information on the training program go to chakradance.com/facilitator-training.

When Natalie's children were young, she began dancing with them. Although Chakradance is only for adults, she could feel that a children's version of Chakradance would truly help to empower young children with life tools and skills. In 2009, Natalie was presented with an opportunity to facilitate a class for children at the wonderful palliative care and respite home, Bear Cottage, in Sydney. Thanks to the beautiful children, parents and staff at Bear Cottage, Chakradance for children took its first steps into the world. But it wasn't until 2013, when Natalie and her husband, Paul, teamed up with Anna Kelly, a holistic therapist, yoga teacher and writer, that Inamojo—a wellbeing program for children—was born. In 2014, they piloted the first series in a primary school in Australia with great success, and classes are now being run across the world. To find information about Inamojo, go to inamojo.com.

Natalie is passionate about how dance, music, mandalas and the chakras help people discover a deeper connection to their true selves and find happier, more balanced lives. She considers this her life's work and continues to develop new workshops and connect with new audiences for both Inamojo and Chakradance.

We hope you enjoyed this Hay House book. If you'd like to receive our online catalog featuring additional information on Hay House books and products, or if you'd like to find out more about the Hay Foundation, please contact:

Hay House, Inc., P.O. Box 5100, Carlsbad, CA 92018-5100
(760) 431-7695 or (800) 654-5126
(760) 431-6948 (fax) or (800) 650-5115 (fax)
www.hayhouse.com® • www.hayfoundation.org

———

Published in Australia by: Hay House Australia Pty. Ltd.,
18/36 Ralph St., Alexandria NSW 2015
Phone: 612-9669-4299 • *Fax:* 612-9669-4144
www.hayhouse.com.au

Published in the United Kingdom by: Hay House UK, Ltd.,
The Sixth Floor, Watson House, 54 Baker Street, London W1U 7BU
Phone: +44 (0)20 3927 7290 • *Fax:* +44 (0)20 3927 7291
www.hayhouse.co.uk

Published in India by: Hay House Publishers India,
Muskaan Complex, Plot No. 3, B-2, Vasant Kunj, New Delhi 110 070
Phone: 91-11-4176-1620 • *Fax:* 91-11-4176-1630
www.hayhouse.co.in

———

Access New Knowledge.
Anytime. Anywhere.

Learn and evolve at your own pace
with the world's leading experts.

www.hayhouseU.com

Printed in the United States
by Baker & Taylor Publisher Services